Alex Hughes @alexskitchenbangers

20 MINUTE LOW-CAL KITCHEN BANGERS

100 super speedy and slimming recipes

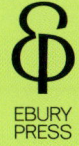

EBURY PRESS

EBURY PRESS

UK | USA | Canada | Ireland | Australia
India | New Zealand | South Africa

Ebury Press is part of the Penguin Random House group of companies whose addresses can be found at global.penguinrandomhouse.com

Penguin Random House UK
One Embassy Gardens, 8 Viaduct Gardens, London SW11 7BW

penguin.co.uk
global.penguinrandomhouse.com

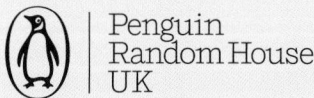

First published by Ebury Press in 2025

2

Copyright © Alex Hughes 2025
Photography © Ellis Parrinder 2025

The moral right of the author has been asserted.

Penguin Random House values and supports copyright. Copyright fuels creativity, encourages diverse voices, promotes freedom of expression and supports a vibrant culture. Thank you for purchasing an authorised edition of this book and for respecting intellectual property laws by not reproducing, scanning or distributing any part of it by any means without permission. You are supporting authors and enabling Penguin Random House to continue to publish books for everyone. No part of this book may be used or reproduced in any manner for the purpose of training artificial intelligence technologies or systems. In accordance with Article 4(3) of the DSM Directive 2019/790, Penguin Random House expressly reserves this work from the text and data mining exception.

Editorial Director: Ru Merritt
Senior Editor: Liv Nightingall
Production Controller: Lucy Harrison
Designer: Nicky Barneby
Photographer: Ellis Parrinder
Food Stylists: Troy Willis and Rosie Reynolds
Prop Stylist: Daisy Shayler-Webb

Colour origination by Altaimage Ltd
Printed and bound in Italy by L.E.G.O. S.p.A.

The authorised representative in the EEA is Penguin Random House Ireland, Morrison Chambers, 32 Nassau Street, Dublin D02 YH68.

A CIP catalogue record for this book is available from the British Library

ISBN 978 152 995605 4

Penguin Random House is committed to a sustainable future for our business, our readers and our planet. This book is made from Forest Stewardship Council® certified paper.

Introduction	4
BRILLIANT BREAKFASTS	6
LUNCHES TO GO	30
LIGHT LUNCHES	48
BATCH COOK	74
DINNERS IN A JIFFY	104
SPEEDY FAKEAWAYS	134
POP IT IN THE PAN	164
Index	190

Introduction

Hey, I'm Alex and I create easy (and banging) low-calorie recipes to help people lose weight.

I created my social media page (@alexskitchenbangers) after navigating a challenging relationship with food over the years. I eventually discovered a healthy way to enjoy the foods I love while losing weight. Starting my Instagram page gave me the opportunity to show people that enjoyment and nourishment – not restriction – are key to a balanced lifestyle.

The problems I hear most from people when it comes to losing weight are:

1. enjoying the food they are eating
2. taking the time out to cook fresh meals.

For this book, I want to make it *even easier* to stick to your weight-loss goals by cutting down the time it takes you to make your meals. All of these recipes take **20 minutes or less** to make. The 20 minutes doesn't include any chopping or prepping, BUT these recipes are so easy that there really isn't much additional prep time involved.

The chapters within this book include **Brilliant Breakfasts, Lunches to Go, Light Lunches, Batch Cook, Dinners in a Jiffy, Speedy Fakeaways** and **Pop it in the Pan**. Whether it's a breakfast burrito bowl to power you through your morning, a BBQ chicken ranch pasta salad for those lunchtime breaks, a baconnaise double cheeseburger to fight off those weekend cravings or a bit of firecracker salmon to spice up those evenings, all of the recipes in this book promise to be quick, nutritious and, most importantly, absolutely banging!

As this book is all about time being of the essence, I've included more **meal-prep recipes** than in my first book, *Low-Cal Kitchen Bangers*. Whenever you are meal prepping food and planning to store it, always make sure that the food is completely cool before placing it in an airtight container in the fridge. I usually use a microwave to reheat my food and do so in one-minute intervals to ensure it doesn't overcook, following the notes below on microwave cooking. Once your food is piping hot, it's good to go! If it is a saucy recipe, you can add a dash of water – or even stock – to help loosen the sauce again.

You will be surprised by how much more quickly you can get meals on the table with just a few tweaks to the way you cook. In this book, there are a few recipes that will require use of a microwave to speed things up a little bit. Please make sure you always use microwavable plates or bowls, rotating them during the cooking if you find your microwave tends to cook unevenly, and use lids to help create steam to lock in moisture, and again, speed up the cooking time. The microwave I use is 1000W. If your microwave wattage is less, a basic formula I like to use to adjust the cooking time is: recipe time x 1000w ÷ by the wattage of your **microwave**. Otherwise, you will find plenty of online converters if you are unsure.

Within the book, I have tried to use most traditional methods of cooking for those of you who do not own an **air fryer**. However, there are a few recipes where I have listed an air fryer as the main cooking method. I've given instructions for an alternative (generally the oven) but the cooking time might be a little longer. For reference, I use an air fryer with an 8.5L capacity that works at between 1450 and 1700 watts. And for those of you who love to use your air fryer all of the time, don't worry, I've also provided the air fryer cooking times for suitable recipes.

Cooking times will always vary depending on the model and make of the appliance you are using. For those of you who prefer to use an oven, or where a recipe indicates for it to be used, the oven I use at home is fan assisted. If you're using a conventional oven, turn up the temperature by 20 degrees or so. I've given you both options on all my recipes and there are plenty of online converters if you are unsure how to adjust your cooking time.

Like my previous book, all of the recipes contain **calorie information** along with a further macro breakdown, including protein, fat and carbohydrate. You'll know if you follow me on social media how important protein is to help with satiety in your diet. For recipes where protein can be increased, I've made sure to add a note for those of you who like to follow a high-protein diet. A lot of my recipes have small quantities in weight (10g for example) rather than tablespoons or teaspoons, as a few grams' difference can alter the calorie count of a recipe significantly. So make sure you invest in some good digital scales to make sure you use the correct measurements!

One other thing you might notice is that since my last book, I've moved away from using low-calorie cooking sprays and now tend to use **olive oil spray** for most recipes. If I have stated 'neutral cooking spray' this refers to a flavourless cooking spray, such as sunflower oil or vegetable oil, as these don't impact the flavour of a dish. Of course, you can use whatever you would prefer.

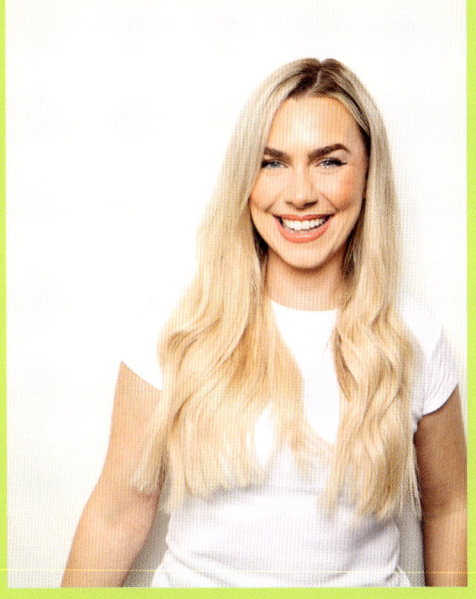

On a final note, I just want to take the time out to thank you for picking up this book. I hope you enjoy everything that you cook from it just as much as I have done writing and creating it. I really love to see everything you make, so please tag me on socials: @alexskitchenbangers

Thank you for the support!

Love,

Alex

RECIPE KEY

 Vegetarian   Dairy free

 Air fryer   Gluten free

 Vegan

One

BRILLIANT BREAKFASTS

Sausage and Egg Muffins

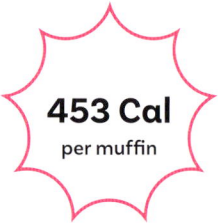

453 Cal per muffin

Protein: 33.6g Fat: 18.8g Carbs: 35.3g

MAKES 4

AF

Snooze that alarm . . . there's no more rushing to eat breakfast in the drive-through when you can make your own banging muffins at home. Breakfast muffins are my fave on-the-go breakfast!

Ingredients

Olive oil spray
8 reduced-fat sausages
1 tsp garlic granules
1 tsp onion granules
1 tsp dried sage
4 medium eggs
4 English muffins
4 light cheese slices
Salt and pepper

Method

- Start by spraying two large frying pans with olive oil spray and leave them over a medium heat.

- Meanwhile, grab the sausages and squeeze the meat from the skins into a bowl. Add the garlic and onion granules and dried sage along with salt and pepper to taste and combine using a fork. Using damp hands, split the mixture into 4 ball-like shapes. Mould into a patty before transferring to one of the hot pans. Repeat with all 4 patties. Flip after 4 minutes, or when browned on the outside, and cook for a further 4 minutes.

- Crack the eggs into the second pan. You can use egg rings to create a circular shape, or use a spatula to push the egg white edges closer to the yolk for the same effect. Fry for 3–4 minutes, or until cooked through. If meal prepping this recipe, you may wish to flip the eggs and cook for a further minute to prevent the yolk leaking.

- While the eggs cook, lightly toast the muffins in a toaster until slightly golden.

- Once the sausage patties are almost cooked, put the cheese slices on top of them. Turn down the heat slightly and leave for a further 2 minutes.

- Grab the toasted muffins and fill with the sausage patties and eggs. If meal prepping the muffins, allow them to cool completely before wrapping tightly. They will store in the fridge for 4–5 days. Alternatively, you can freeze them for up to 3 months; simply defrost 24 hours prior to when you wish to eat them, then microwave in a damp piece of kitchen paper in 30-second intervals until piping throughout. Alternatively, you can pop them in the oven at 200°C/180°C fan for 8–10 minutes.

Air fryer You can cook the sausage patties in the air fryer at 190°C for 3–4 minutes.

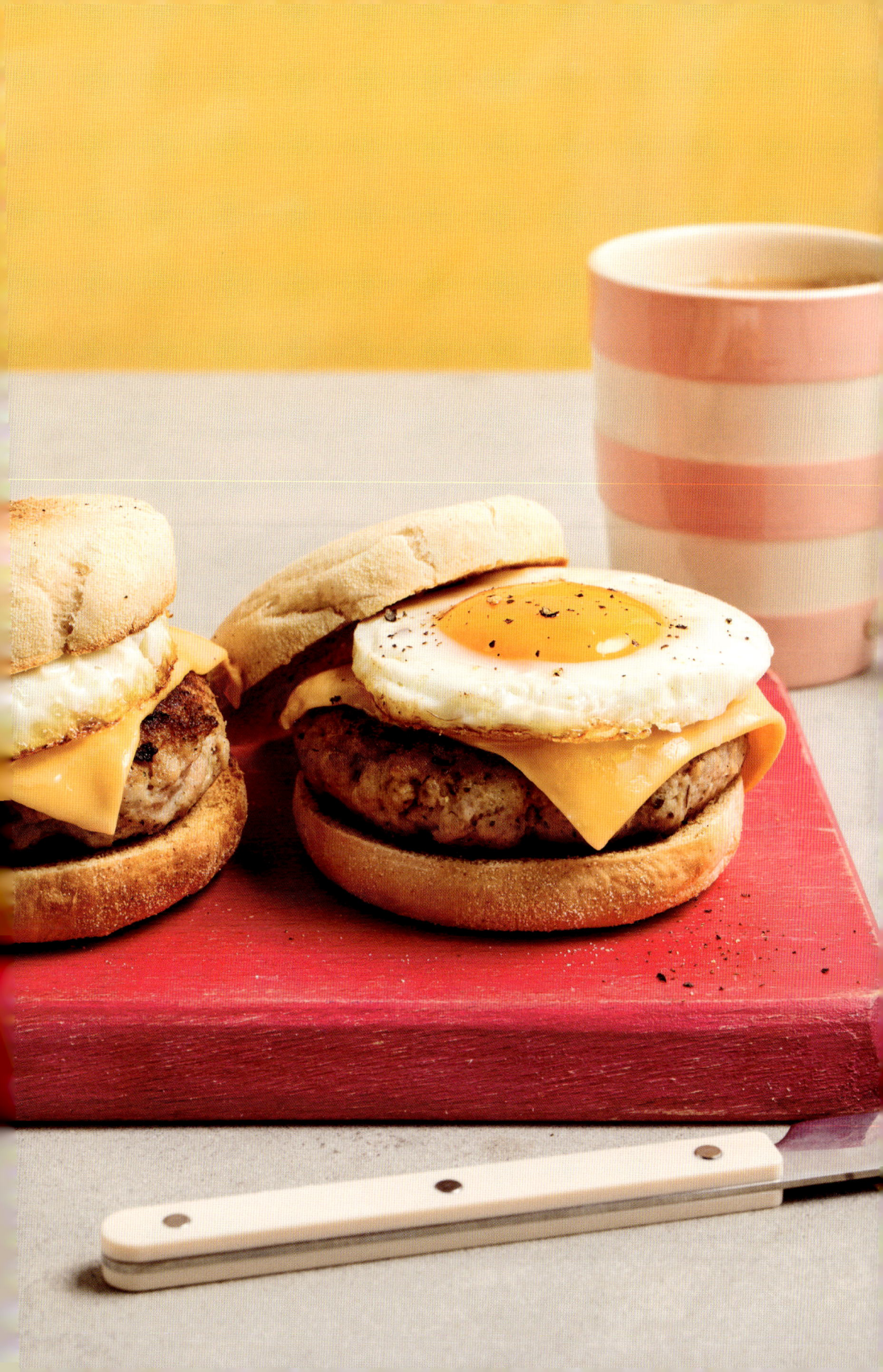

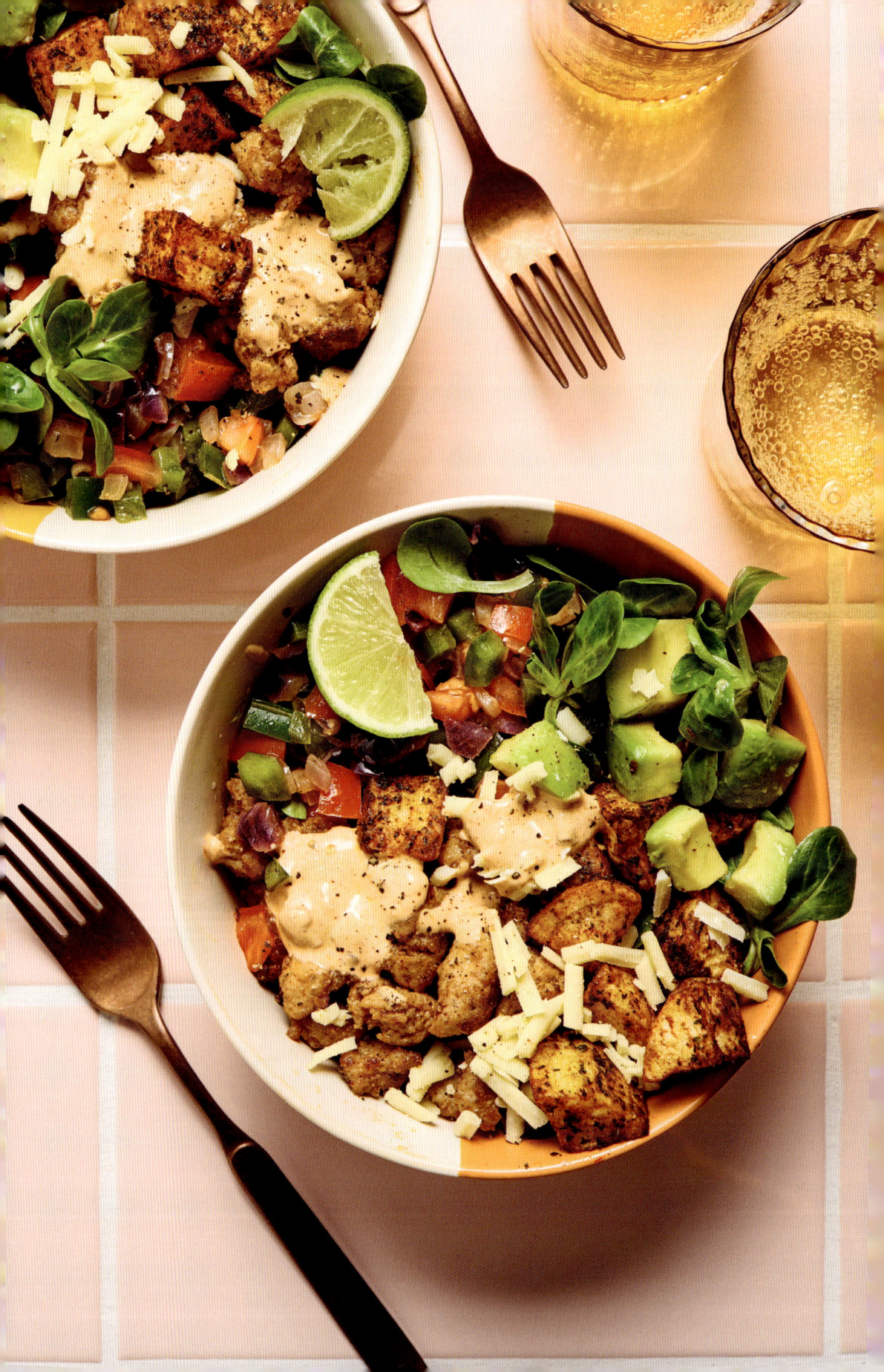

Breakfast Burrito Bowls

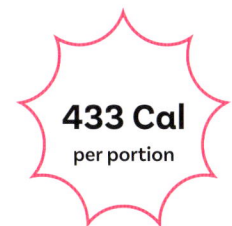

433 Cal per portion

Protein: 26.4g   Fat: 18.3g   Carbs: 35.2g

SERVES 2

 AF

This is an absolute banger. If you can't get lamb's lettuce, sub it for some spinach. To boost the protein, opt for chicken chipolatas or add some scrambled egg, and to make this dish vegetarian, opt for meat-free sausages.

Ingredients

250g Maris Piper potato, peeled and cut into 2cm cubes

1 tsp smoked paprika

1 tsp dried parsley

Olive oil spray

4 reduced-fat pork sausages

1 tsp taco seasoning

50ml water

1 small green pepper, finely diced

1 small red onion, finely diced

1 large salad tomato, diced

40g lamb's lettuce

50g avocado, cubed

20g reduced-fat cheddar, grated

Sauce

50g fat-free Greek yoghurt

½ tsp chipotle paste

1 tsp lime juice

Salt

Method

- Start by patting the potato dry with kitchen paper and placing it directly into the air fryer drawer. Season with the smoked paprika and parsley along with some salt and pepper. Shake well to distribute the seasonings, spray with a few pumps of olive oil spray and air fry for 17 minutes at 200°C shaking every 5 minutes or so.

- Next, add a few pumps of olive oil spray to a large frying pan. Squeeze the sausages out of their skins directly into the pan. Fry over a high heat, breaking the meat into smaller pieces. Cook for 7 minutes or so, until browned.

- While the sausage meat cooks, prepare the sauce by mixing together all the ingredients and set to one side.

- Once the sausage meat has browned, add the taco seasoning, mixing well to combine, and then pour in the water. Mix for a further minute and remove from the pan.

- Add the pepper, onion and tomato to the same pan. Sauté for a minute or two until they have slightly softened, then take off the stove.

- While the potatoes finish cooking, build the bowls. First put in the lettuce, followed by the veggies, sausage meat, avocado, grated cheddar and finally the cooked potatoes.

- Finish by drizzling over the sauce.

Oven For the potatoes, place them directly onto a baking tray. Cook for 20–25 minutes at the same temperature, tossing regularly throughout.

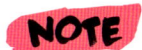

If meal prepping, add the lettuce and avocado fresh.

Eggcado Breakfast Sandwiches

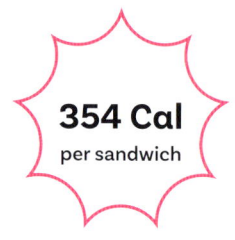

354 Cal per sandwich

| Protein: 18.3g | Fat: 16.9g | Carbs: 30.9g |

MAKES 2

Start your day in a delicious way with these gorgeous egg sandwiches. Boiled eggs are mixed with mayonnaise, spring onion and sriracha to create an egg salad that's paired with avocado, tomato and spinach for a banging breakfast. If you plan to prepare this recipe ahead of time to eat on the go, opt to stuff the mix into soft pitta breads or toasted sourdough to hold the filling.

Ingredients

4 medium eggs
2 brioche buns
25g lighter than light mayonnaise
10g sriracha sauce
1 spring onion, sliced
15g baby spinach
40g avocado, sliced
1 salad tomato, thinly sliced
Salt and pepper

Method

- Start by adding the eggs to a large pan of boiling water. Leave to cook over a high heat for 8 minutes.
- Meanwhile, toast the brioche buns until golden.
- Once the egg timer is up, transfer the eggs to an ice bath for 3 minutes. Remove from the bath, crack the shells using a knife and peel the eggs, transferring them to a bowl.
- To the same bowl, add the light mayo and 1 teaspoon of the sriracha sauce. Season with salt and pepper before folding in the spring onion and breaking up the egg into smaller pieces.
- Put the spinach onto each of the bottom buns, then top with the egg salad mix, the sliced avocado, then the tomato, and finish by drizzling over the remaining sriracha sauce.

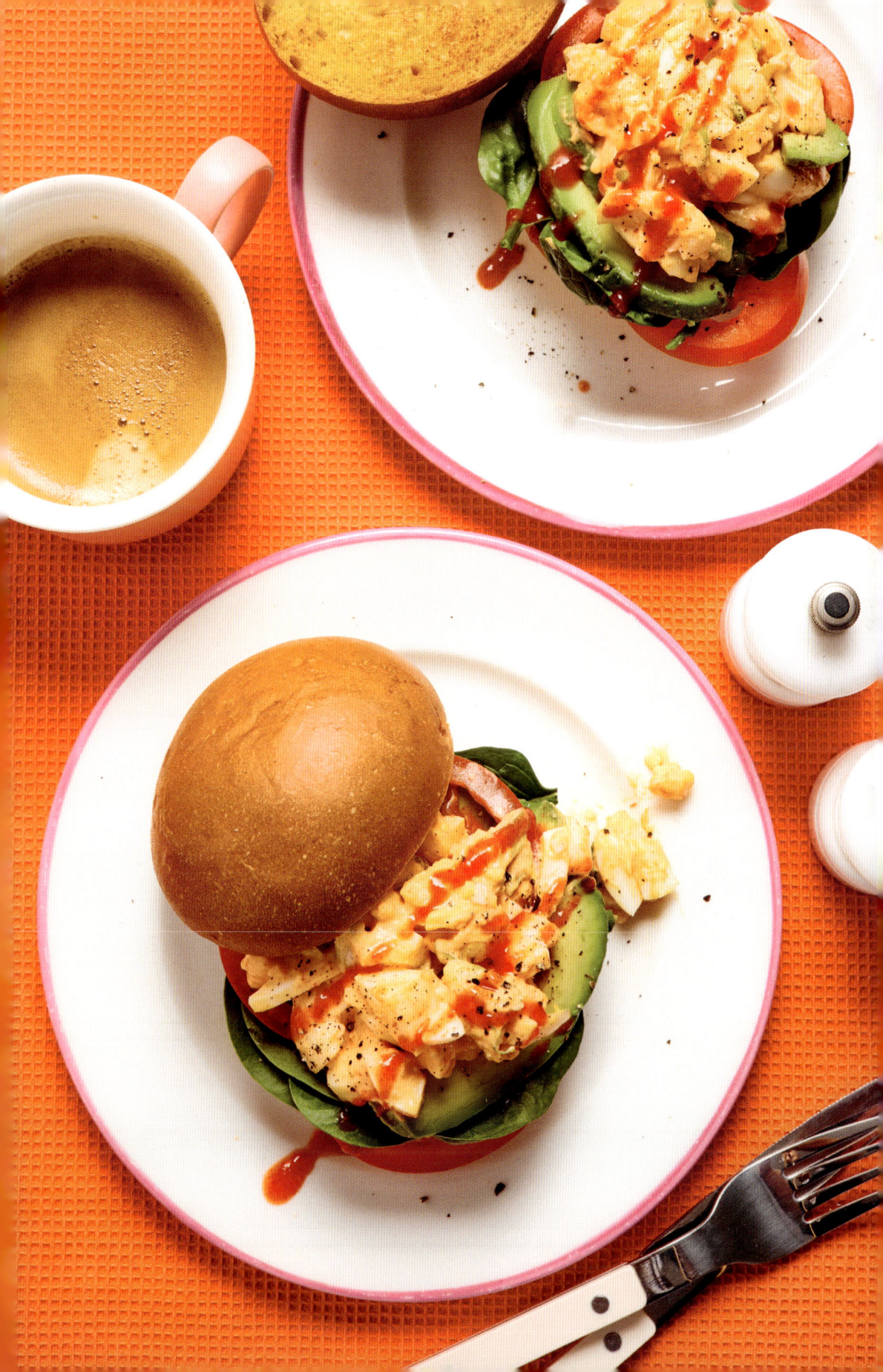

Smashed Sausage Tacos

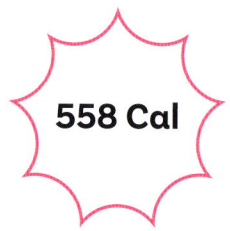

Protein: 34.2g **Fat: 29.5g** **Carbs: 37.3g**

SERVES 1

Say hello to the speediest and tastiest breakfast. Pork sausages are smashed onto flour tortillas and fried until they are super crispy. Paired with egg and avo this is a breakfast you will smash on repeat. Feel free to switch it up and use chicken chipolatas or turkey sausages for a lighter bite.

Ingredients

Olive oil spray
2 reduced-fat pork sausages
2 mini tortilla wraps
2 medium eggs, whisked
30g ripe avocado
10g chilli jam
1 spring onion, sliced
Salt and pepper

Method

- Start by spraying one large and one small frying pan with olive oil spray and leave each over medium heat.
- Squeeze the sausage meat out of the skins directly onto the wraps. Using a fork, smash down the meat to cover the surface of the wraps. Season with salt and pepper to taste.
- Transfer the wraps to the large pan, meat-side down, and cook for 7 minutes over a medium heat.
- Meanwhile, add the whisked eggs to the other pan. Over a low heat, leave the eggs to set, then gently fold inwards to scramble. Split into two and remove the pan from the heat. You want the eggs slightly underdone, as they will continue to cook in the heat of the pan.
- In a bowl, smash the avocado using a fork. Season with a pinch of salt.
- Once the 7 minutes is up, flip the wraps for a further minute. Remove from the heat and top with the smashed avocado, eggs, chilli jam and fresh spring onion.

Spinach, Egg and Feta Wrap

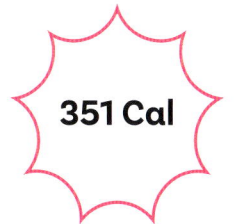

351 Cal

Protein: 28.3g Fat: 10g Carbs: 34.7g

MAKES 1

This is one of my new favourite go-tos for breakfast. It's a dupe for one you can get in a large coffee branch (ahem) and it is one you can easily take on the go. The sun-dried tomatoes bring this wrap to life but you can swap them out for cherry tomatoes if you wish, and while egg whites give this wrap a protein boost while minimising calories, you can simply swap for 3 medium eggs.

Ingredients

Olive oil spray
Handful of spinach, chopped
20g sun-dried tomatoes, chopped
150g egg whites
½ tsp Italian herb seasoning
30g lightest cream cheese
1 tortilla wrap
20g feta, chopped
Salt and pepper

Method

- Start by spraying a medium frying pan with olive oil spray. Over a medium heat, add the spinach and sun-dried tomatoes and fry for a couple of minutes, until the spinach has wilted slightly.
- Once the spinach has wilted, add the egg whites and herb seasoning. Season with salt and pepper to taste.
- Fry for 3-4 minutes, until the egg whites have set. Fold the eggs in half and then half again. Remove from the pan.
- Spread the cream cheese in the centre of the wrap. Top with the egg quarter and the crumbled feta.
- Fold the inside of the wrap into the centre, then roll, tucking in edges as you fold, into a burrito shape.
- Add the wrap back into the same pan for a minute each side until toasted.
- Slice and serve.

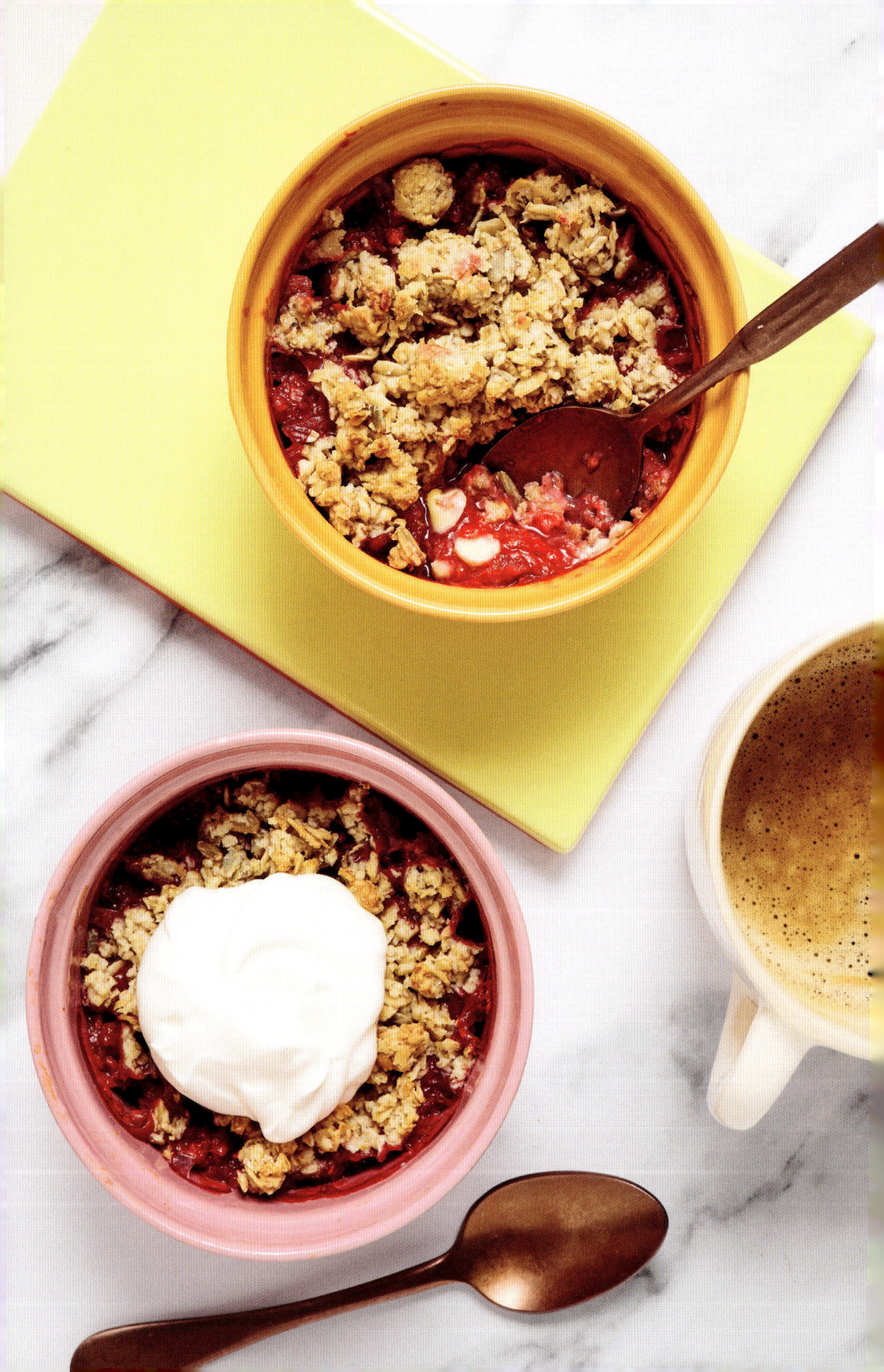

White Chocolate Raspberry Breakfast Crumble

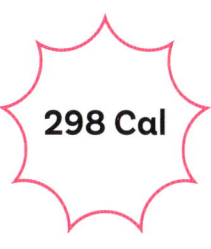 298 Cal

Protein: 6.3g Fat: 10.7g Carbs: 45.7g

SERVES 1

Did someone say dessert for breakfast? That's cheeky, but absolutely guilt free with this fruit-packed crumble. You can sub the raspberries for any frozen fruit you like if they aren't your jam. For an added protein boost, omit the plain flour and add a scoop of vanilla protein powder.

Ingredients

100g frozen raspberries
13g plain flour
1 tsp lemon juice
30g rolled oats
10g light butter, at room temperature
1 tbsp granulated sweetener
1 tbsp skimmed milk
5g white chocolate chips
1 tbsp plain or vanilla fat-free Greek yoghurt, to serve

Method

- Preheat the oven to 210°C/190°C fan.
- Start by putting the raspberries into an ovenproof bowl (I use 400ml capacity for this recipe – you want to ensure it has a wide surface for everything to cook quicker). Toss the raspberries with ¼ teaspoon of the flour before drizzling over the lemon juice. Cook in the microwave on high for a minute.
- Meanwhile, in a bowl, mix together the oats, the remaining 10g plain flour, the butter, sweetener and milk. Use your fingertips to rub the mixture together and create a crumbly texture.
- Scatter the white chocolate chips over the raspberries, followed by the crumble mix, covering the surface. Return to the microwave for 1 minute.
- Remove from the microwave and place in the oven for 12 minutes, then remove and serve with the yoghurt on top.

Air fryer At step 5, put the crumble dish into the air fryer basket for 8 minutes at 170°C.

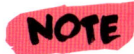

You could make a larger batch of this recipe and store it in the fridge for up to 4 days.

Full English Shakshuka

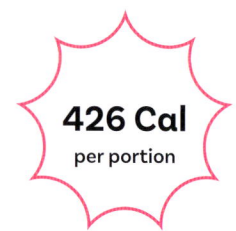
426 Cal per portion

| Protein: 33.3g | Fat: 16.5g | Carbs: 23.5g |

SERVES 2

The perfect weekend brunch recipe has arrived. Shakshuka recipes have been a staple in my weight loss journey and what better way to serve it than by cranking it up full English style. This recipe is full of protein and veggies to help keep you feeling full and satisfied. Best served with some golden sourdough for dipping.

Ingredients

4 reduced-fat pork sausages
Olive oil spray
150g mushrooms, sliced
1 white onion, diced
1 tsp chopped garlic
1 × 400g tin of chopped tomatoes
20g reduced-sugar ketchup
118g tinned haricot beans (½ tin)
50ml water
½ tsp chilli flakes (optional)
1 tsp paprika
2 bacon medallions
2 medium eggs
Salt and pepper
A couple of sprigs of fresh parsley, to garnish

Method

- Start by preheating the grill to medium and cooking the sausages for 16 minutes, turning occasionally (please check the packet instructions for full cooking times).
- Next, spray a medium frying pan with olive oil spray. Add the mushrooms and fry over a high heat for 3–4 minutes, until golden, then remove from the pan and set aside.
- Next, add the onion and garlic and fry for 1 minute, continuously moving them around.
- Remove from the hob and pour in the chopped tomatoes, then add the ketchup and haricot beans. Pour the water into the tomato tin, swirl it around and empty into the pan. Return the mushrooms to the pan over a medium-high heat.
- Season the dish with the chilli flakes, if using; add the paprika and salt and pepper to taste and leave for 2 minutes to bubble.
- While the dish bubbles, put the bacon under the grill along with the sausages and cook for 5–7 minutes, or until cooking to your liking. Once cooked, cut into strips.
- Next, make two wells in the tomatoes, crack the eggs into the wells, then cover the pan and leave over a medium–low heat for around 5 minutes, until the egg whites are set.
- Once the egg whites are set, nestle the sausage into the pan along with the cut bacon.
- Finish by garnishing with the parsley.

Air fryer Most sausages can be air fried if you prefer. Place in a preheated air fryer basket at 180°C for 12 minutes. Bacon can be cooked at the same temperature for 6–8 minutes, turning part-way through.

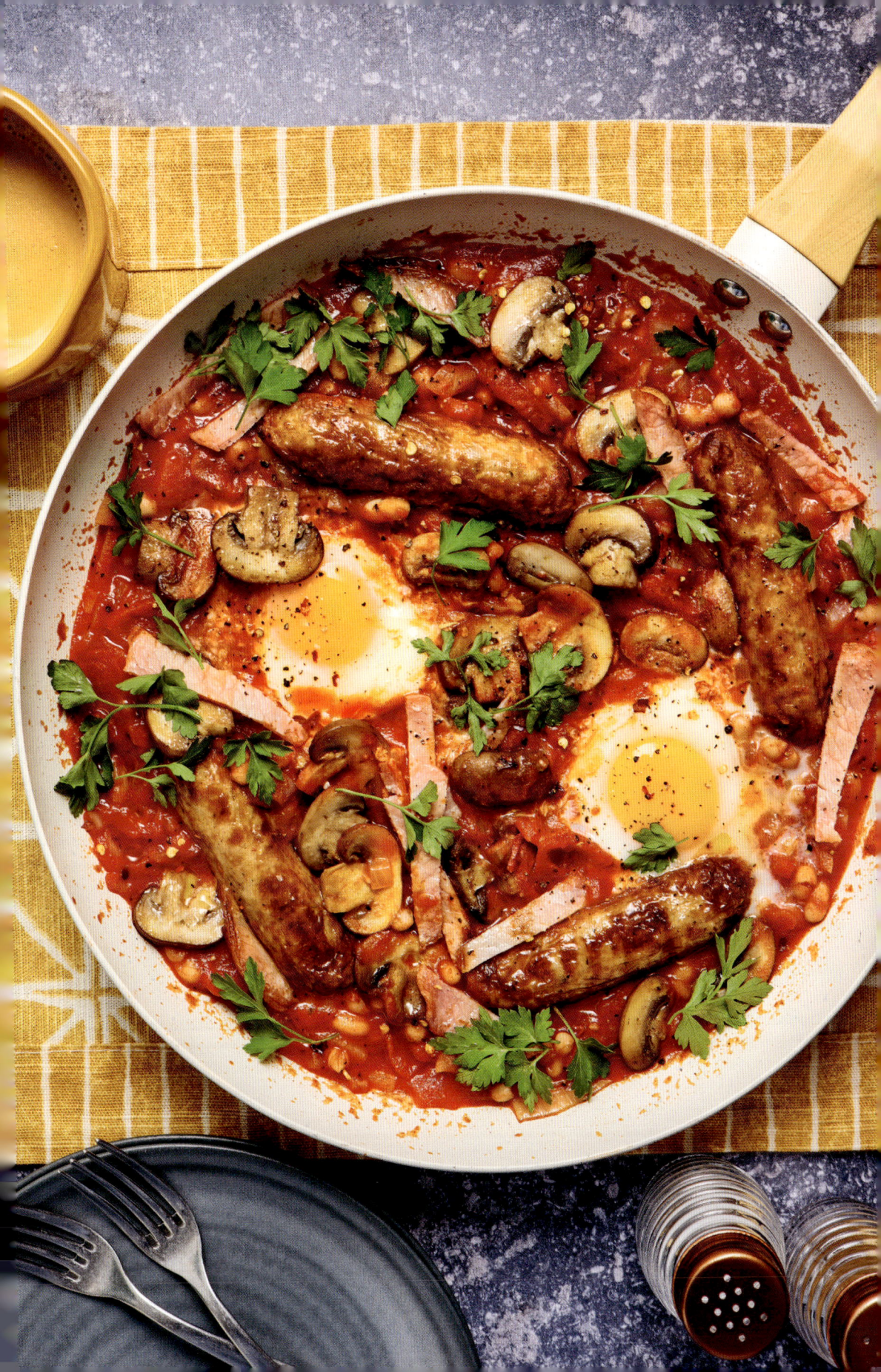

Lightened-Up Hollandaise Sauce Over Eggs

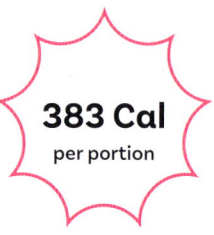

383 Cal per portion

`Protein: 20.2g` `Fat: 18.2g` `Carbs: 33g`

SERVES 2

Usually considered an indulgent breakfast, this lightened-up version of hollandaise sauce is the answer to your weight-loss prayers.

Ingredients

1 tbsp distilled white vinegar
4 medium eggs
2 English muffins
2 chives, chopped

Hollandaise sauce

1 medium egg yolk
60g fat-free Greek yoghurt
½ tsp lemon juice
¼ tsp Dijon mustard (or mustard powder)
1 tsp cornflour
20g light butter
Salt and pepper

Method

- Start by heating 2.5cm of water in a medium saucepan. Sit a bowl big enough to cover the pan on top, or place a sieve on top, then sit a smaller bowl inside it.
- Put the egg yolk, yoghurt, lemon juice and mustard into the bowl. Whisk well and leave over a medium heat for 10 minutes. Intermittently lift the bowl to allow the steam to escape.
- Once the 10 minutes is up, stir in the cornflour and turn the heat down to low.
- Next, fill a large saucepan with hot water and add the vinegar. Bring to a boil.
- Once it starts to boil, turn down the heat to a simmer whereby only small bubbles rise to the surface.
- Crack the eggs into a bowl. Stir the water in the pan to create a whirlpool. Carefully slide each egg into the water, ensuring there is enough room for all the eggs; if not, do two at a time. Cook for 4 minutes or until the egg white has set. Once set, carefully remove from the pan using a slotted spoon and place on kitchen paper to absorb any excess water.
- While the eggs cook, lightly toast each muffin.
- Top the muffins with the eggs.
- Remove the hollandaise sauce from the heat, stir through the butter and season with salt and pepper. You should have a nice thick sauce. If you need a thicker sauce, you can put all of the sauce directly into the pan over a medium heat and whisk for a minute (but no longer than this) to prevent the yoghurt from curdling.
- Serve the sauce over the muffins, garnishing with the chives.

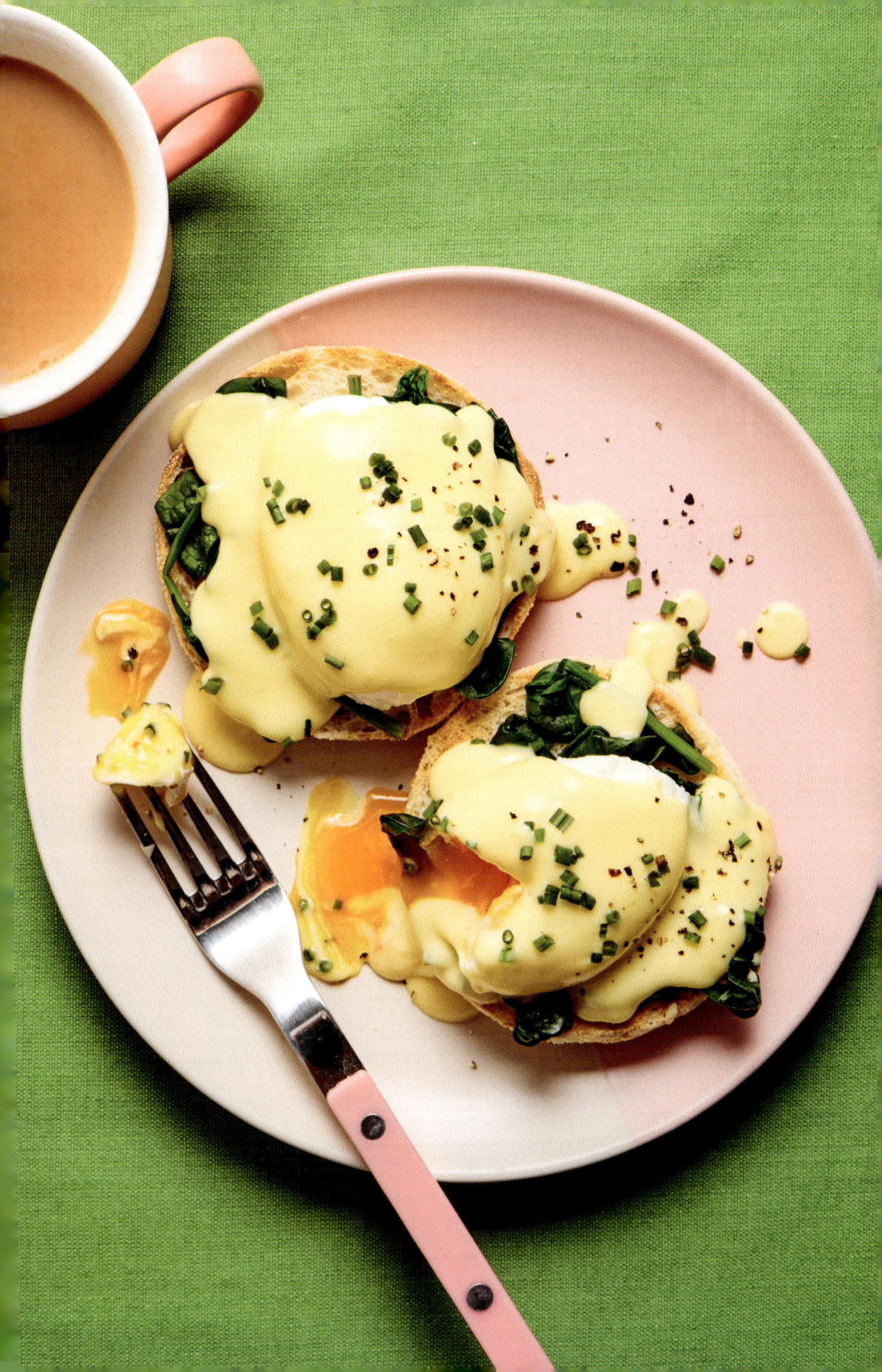

Banoffee Pie Pancake Stack

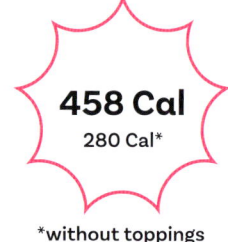

458 Cal
280 Cal*

*without toppings

| Protein: 13.4g / 9.3g* | Fat: 8.5g / 5.9g* | Carbs: 76.3g / 41.1g* |

SERVES 1

Okay, these are an 'indulgent' breakfast but sometimes you just need the full works to power you through your day. These pancakes are stacked with sliced banana, caramel sauce, a dollop of yoghurt and a biscuit to give the flavours of a banoffee pie. I've listed the macros without the toppings if you wish to play around with your own.

Ingredients

50g plain flour
1 tbsp granulated sweetener
¼ tsp salt
½ tsp baking powder
1 medium egg
40ml skimmed milk
15g fat-free Greek yoghurt
1 tsp vanilla extract
Olive oil spray

For the topping

1 small banana, sliced
15g caramel sauce (I use Carnation's Caramel Drizzle Sauce)
15g fat-free Greek yoghurt
1 caramelised biscuit, crumbled

Method

- Start by sifting the plain flour into a bowl. Add the granulated sweetener, salt and baking powder and mix well.
- Next, combine the egg, milk, yoghurt and vanilla extract in a separate bowl. Fold the wet ingredients into the dry, mixing until just combined – do not overmix.
- Leave to one side while you preheat a large frying pan over a medium heat. Spray with a few pumps of olive oil spray.
- Add 2 tablespoons of batter per pancake to the frying pan. The mixture should make 4 in total. Leave for a couple of minutes until bubbles start to appear on the top.
- Using a spatula, carefully lift to check the underneath is golden prior to flipping. Flip and cook for another 2-3 minutes, until golden on the bottom side.
- Remove the pancakes from the pan. Top a pancake with slices of banana, then cover with another pancake and another layer of banana, reserving some banana to finish. On the top pancake, drizzle over the caramel sauce, then top with the remaining banana, the yoghurt and crumbled biscuit.

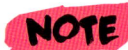

You can store the cooked pancakes (without the toppings) in the fridge for up to 4 days. Reheat in the microwave for 15-30 seconds. If you want to add protein powder, replace 20g of the flour with 20g vanilla protein powder. You may need to add a touch more milk.

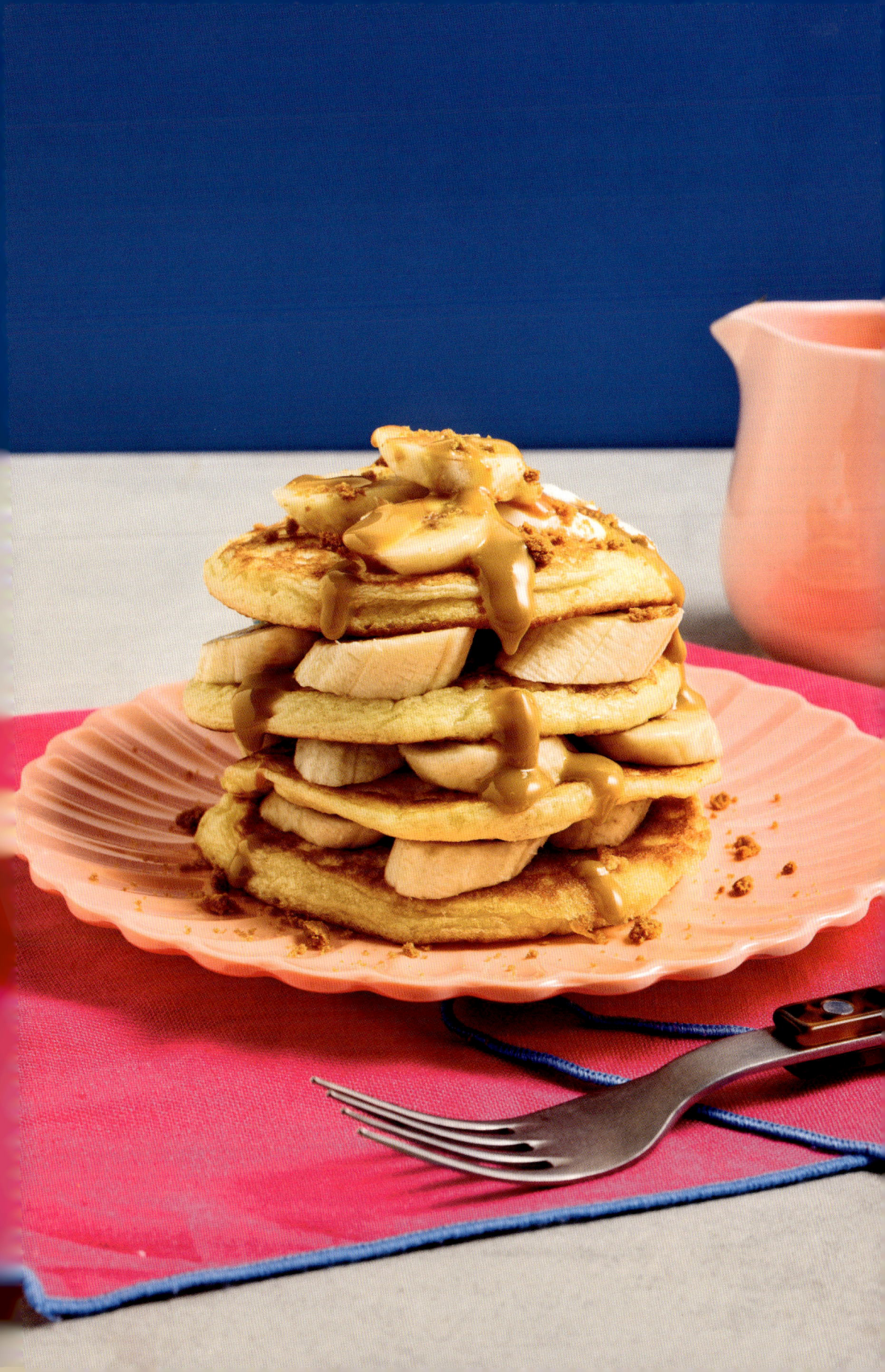

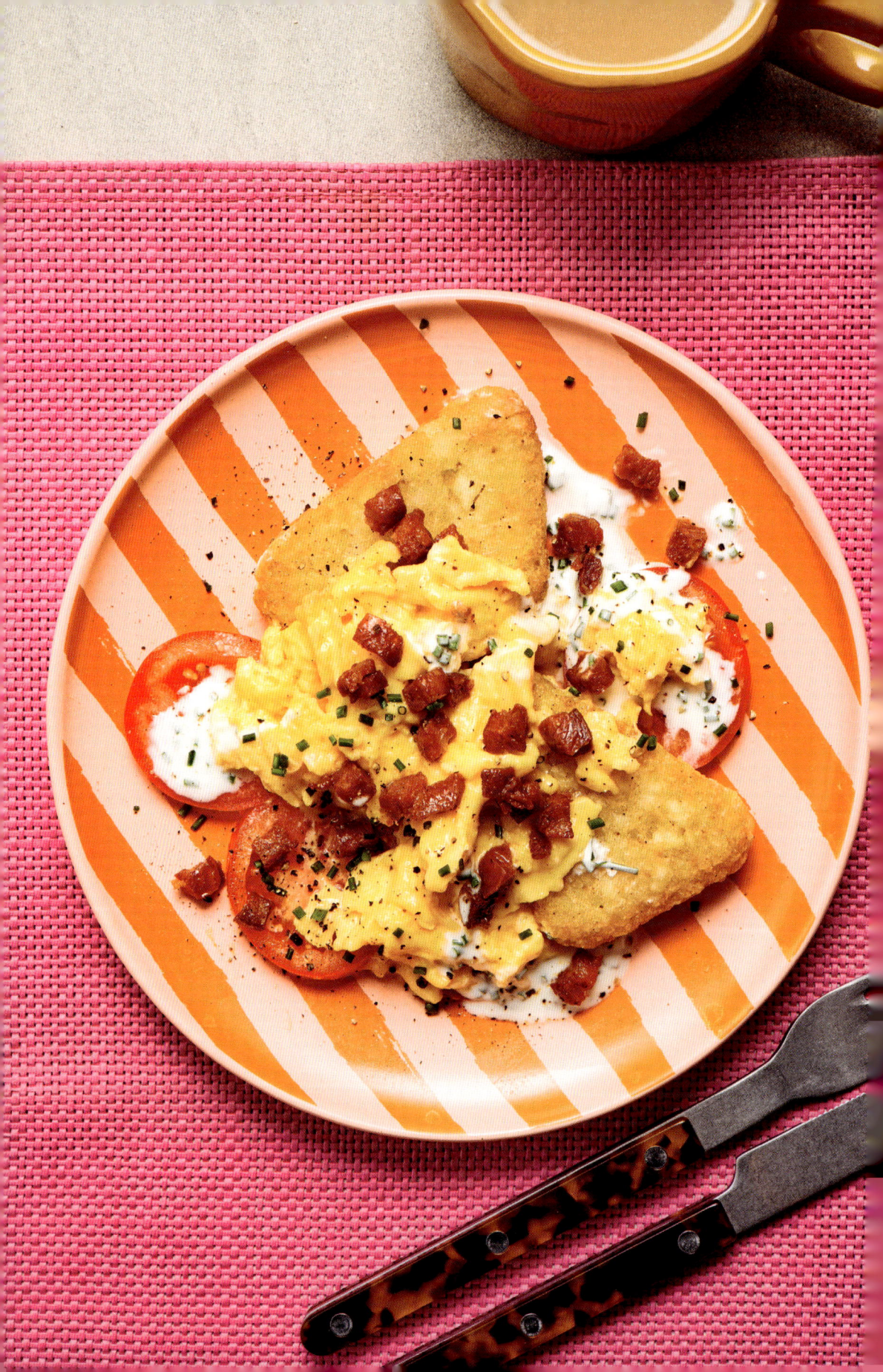

Loaded Egg and Chorizo Hash Browns

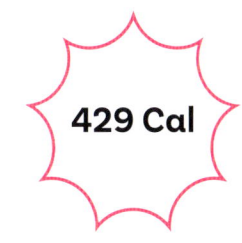

Protein: 19.9g   **Fat: 24.7g**   **Carbs: 27.7g**

SERVES 1

There is no better way to start the day than with a crispy hash brown, especially loaded ones. This version has a yoghurt chive sauce, juicy sliced tomato, scrambled egg, and is finished with crispy chorizo. You can replace the chorizo with lean bacon or sausage if you wish.

Ingredients

2 hash browns (I use the ones from Aldi)
15g chorizo, diced
2 medium eggs
5g butter
1 vine tomato, sliced
Salt and pepper
2 chives (can sub for ¼ tsp dried), chopped, to garnish

Chive sauce

30g fat-free Greek yoghurt
⅛ tsp garlic granules
⅛ tsp onion granules
4 chives, chopped (can sub for ½ tsp dried)
1 tsp distilled white vinegar

Method

- Start by cooking the hash browns according to the packet instructions (I usually air fry mine for 14 minutes at 195°C).
- While the hash browns cook, make the chive sauce by stirring all the ingredients together and then set to one side.
- When there's around 10 minutes left on the hash browns, add the diced chorizo to a frying pan. Fry over a high heat for 3-4 minutes, until crispy, then remove from the pan, leaving the oils behind.
- Next, whisk the eggs in a jug, seasoning with salt and pepper.
- Turn the heat under the pan down to low, pour in the eggs and leave to set for a minute. Then add the butter before folding to scramble. Remove the eggs from the heat just before they look cooked, as they will continue to cook off the hob.
- Once everything is ready, first layer the chive sauce on top of the hash browns, followed by the sliced tomato, scrambled egg, and crispy chorizo, and garnish with the chopped chives.

Scrambled Oat Bowl

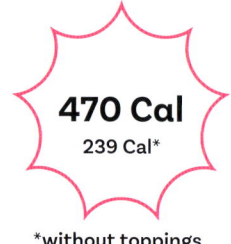

470 Cal
239 Cal*

*without toppings

| Protein: 33g / 12.6g* | Fat: 14.1g / 8.4g* | Carbs: 44.1g / 22.5g* |

SERVES 1

I love a good viral recipe, especially when it's a breakfast one. If you've not tried this before, a quick oat mixture is made and then pan-fried to create what resembles crispy yet soft bites of 'granola'. I've put my own twist on it, creating a recipe without bananas. If you've got a bit of a sweet tooth, feel free to add more sweetener, swap to honey for a natural alternative, or add a teaspoon of cocoa powder for a chocolate version.

Ingredients

40g rolled oats
1 tbsp granulated sweetener
1 medium egg
20g fat-free Greek yoghurt
10ml semi-skimmed milk
Olive oil spray

To serve
200g vanilla yoghurt
80g strawberries, sliced
10g peanut butter

Method

- Start by adding the oats to a bowl. Sprinkle in the sweetener before adding the egg, yoghurt and milk. Stir to combine.
- Next, set a frying pan over a medium heat. Spray with a few pumps of olive oil spray, then add the oat mixture in a similar shape to a large pancake.
- Leave undisturbed for a minute and a half, until browned underneath, then flip and cook for the same amount of time.
- Start to break up into smaller pieces until the mix resembles clusters.
- Turn the heat up slightly for a few more minutes to make the oats golden and crisp, then remove the pan from the hob.
- Put the vanilla yoghurt into a bowl, along with the oat clusters and strawberries.
- In a microwavable bowl, blast the peanut butter in the microwave on high for 15-20 seconds, until slightly runny. Drizzle over the oat bowl before serving.

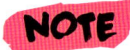

If you do like banana, you can use 80g of banana in place of the yoghurt, milk and sweetener.

'On the Go' Omelette

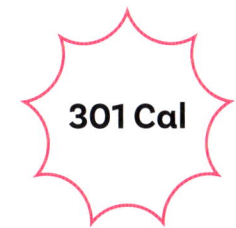

301 Cal

Protein: 30.5g **Fat: 18g** **Carbs: 3.8g**

SERVES 1

If you're the kind of person that's running out the door while still putting your shoes on in the morning, I have got you covered with this breakfast recipe. Add all of the usual omelette ingredients to a container and when you get to work, simply microwave for a few minutes and you'll have yourself a satisfying breakfast. This is of course a super-versatile recipe so play around with the ingredients and what suits your palate.

Ingredients

Olive oil spray
5 cherry tomatoes, quartered
2 spring onions, diced
50g ham, chopped
20g reduced-fat cheddar, grated
½ tsp garlic granules
5g light butter
2 medium eggs, whisked
Salt and pepper

Method

- Start by spraying a 400ml round microwavable container with olive oil spray.
- Next, add the cherry tomatoes, spring onions, ham and cheese. Season with salt, pepper and the garlic granules before tossing together with a spoon.
- Add the butter and eggs. Use the lid to cover before giving everything a good shake.
- When ready to heat, remove the lid and place the container in the microwave. Cook on high, initially for 1 minute, then give it a good stir and blast it for a further minute. Keep blasting in 20-second intervals until the middle is no longer runny. Depending on your microwave (see page 4) this might be for up to a couple of minutes.
- Once the centre is no longer runny, carefully remove from the microwave and leave to stand for a minute before eating.

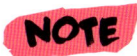

Do not add the eggs if prepping for the following day, as they won't stay fresh.

Chocolate Chip Brioche French Toast Bites

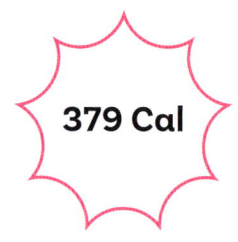

379 Cal

| Protein: 13.8g | Fat: 14.6g | Carbs: 43.3g |

SERVES 1

For those who have a sweet tooth, this breakfast will answer all of your prayers. Chocolate chip brioche rolls are my favourite way to make French toast bites because the chocolate inside melts while being pan-fried. You can use any fruit you like to top these bites and for an added protein boost, you can add half a scoop of protein powder to the egg and milk mixture.

Ingredients

2 chocolate chip brioche rolls
1 small egg
40ml semi-skimmed milk
Neutral cooking spray
50g frozen raspberries
¼ tsp icing sugar
5g liquid chocolate (I use Sweet Freedom)
20g fat-free Greek yoghurt

Method

- Start by slicing the brioche rolls in half. Cut into small squares and set to one side.
- Next, add the egg and milk to a small bowl and whisk until well combined.
- Heat a large pan over a medium heat and spray with a few pumps of cooking spray. Dip each bit of brioche into the egg mix before popping into the pan.
- Pan-fry all sides of the square for around a minute each until toasted and golden. Remove from the pan and transfer to a bowl.
- Top the bites with the raspberries, then sprinkle over the icing sugar. Drizzle over the liquid chocolate before dolloping on the Greek yoghurt.

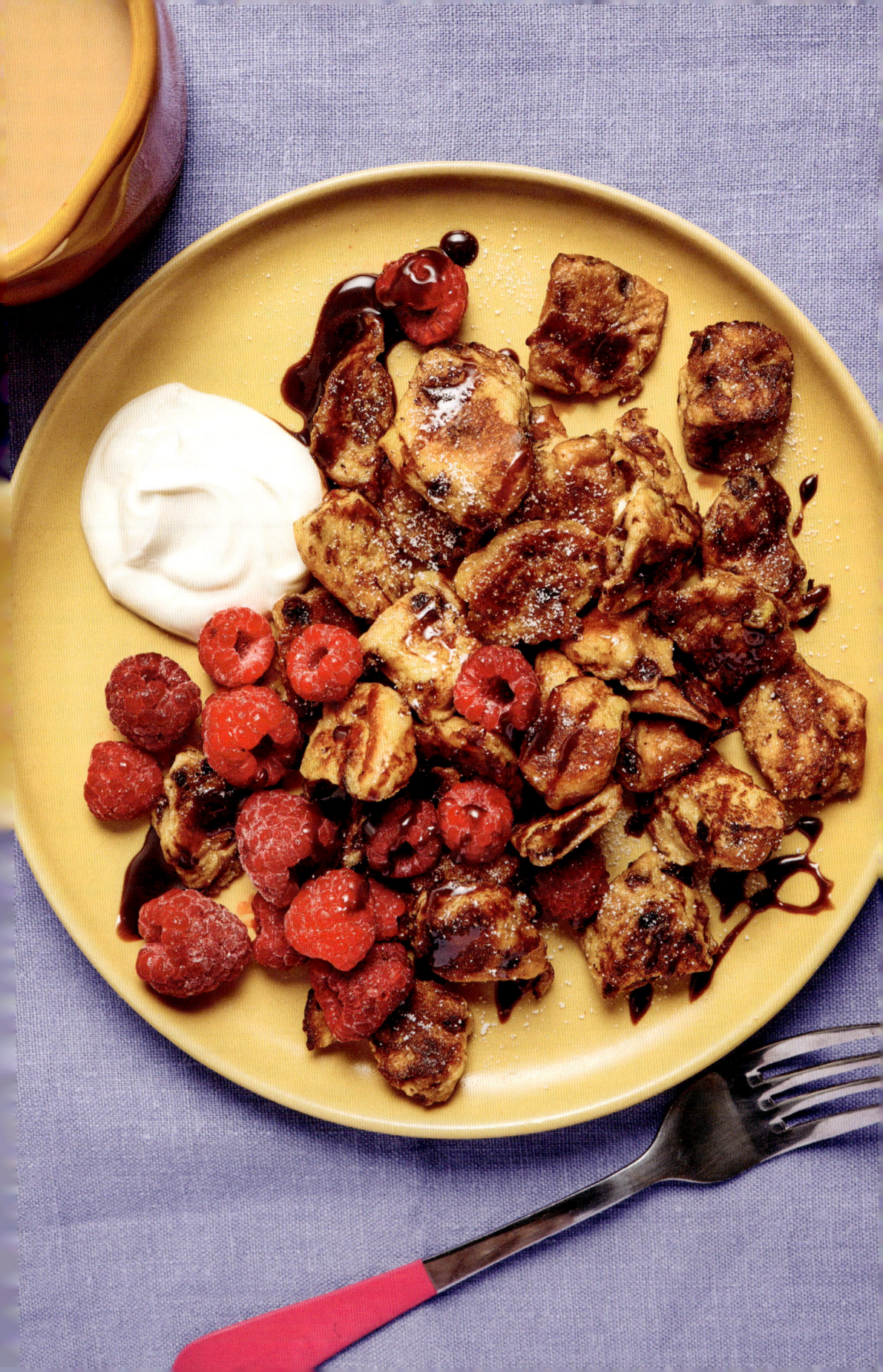

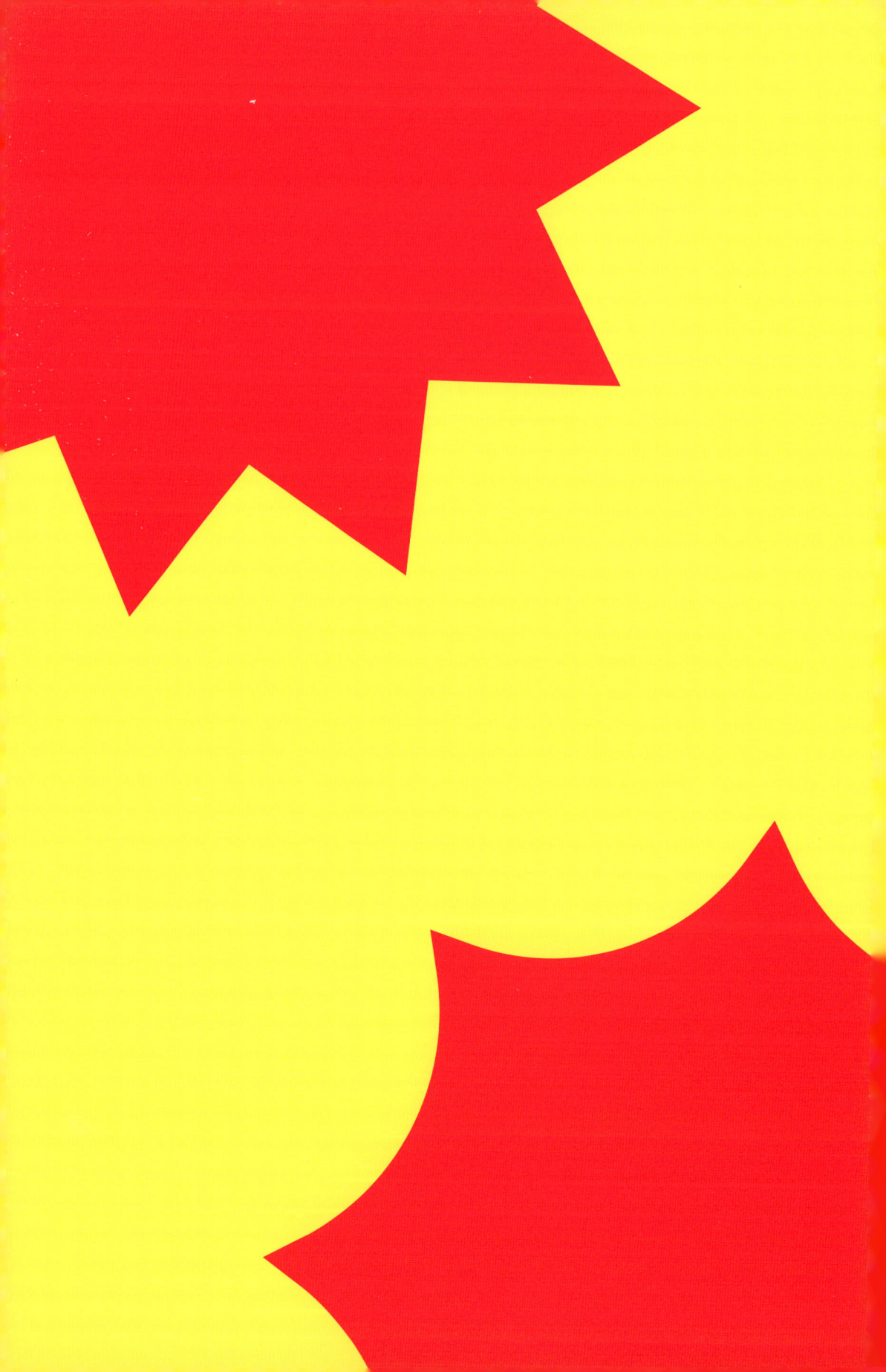

Two

LUNCHES TO GO

BBQ Chicken Ranch Pasta Salad

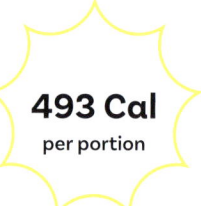

493 Cal per portion

Protein: 42.7g **Fat: 11.6g** **Carbs: 49.7g**

SERVES 2

This is one of those recipes that's healthy but definitely tantalises the taste buds. It's packed full of flavour thanks to the seasoned barbecue chicken bites and yoghurt ranch sauce. Feel free to swap the salad items for any you like.

Ingredients

100g dried pasta

200g skinless chicken breast, cut into 2.5cm cubes

1½ tsp barbecue seasoning

Olive oil spray

15g ranch dressing

100g fat-free Greek yoghurt

10g barbecue sauce

1 tbsp water

80g lettuce, shredded

40g sweetcorn

1 small red onion, diced

3 salad tomatoes, chopped

20g Red Leicester, grated (can sub for reduced-fat cheddar)

1 tsp bacon bits

Method

- Start by putting the pasta into a large pan of salted boiling water. Cook according to the packet instructions, until al dente. Once cooked, drain and rinse with cold water.
- Next, dust the chicken all over with the barbecue seasoning.
- Spray a large frying pan with a few pumps of olive oil spray. Add the chicken to the pan and cook over a medium-high heat for 8 minutes or until cooked through.
- While the chicken cooks, mix together the ranch dressing and Greek yoghurt and set to one side.
- When the chicken is cooked, squeeze in the barbecue sauce along with the tablespoon of water to loosen. Toss to combine and leave to one side to cool slightly.
- To a large bowl, add the shredded lettuce, cooked pasta, sweetcorn, red onion, tomatoes, grated cheese and bacon bits. Top with the cooled chicken.
- Toss with the ranch sauce until all of the ingredients are fully combined.

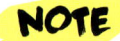

When meal prepping pasta salads, wait for the pasta and chicken to cool completely before popping them in an airtight container. If you are able to, store the lettuce in a sandwich bag to prevent it from going brown and add it fresh when eating.

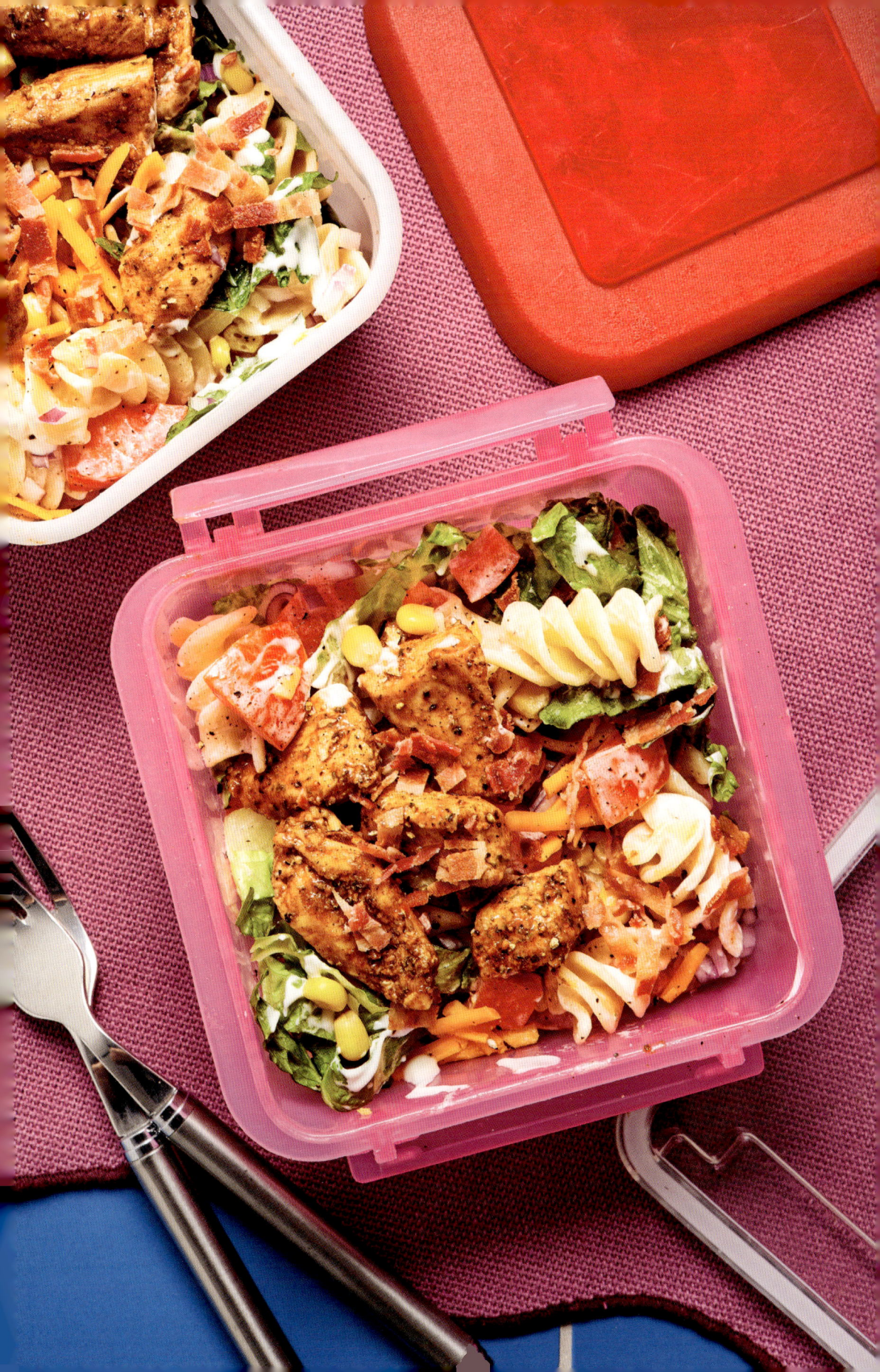

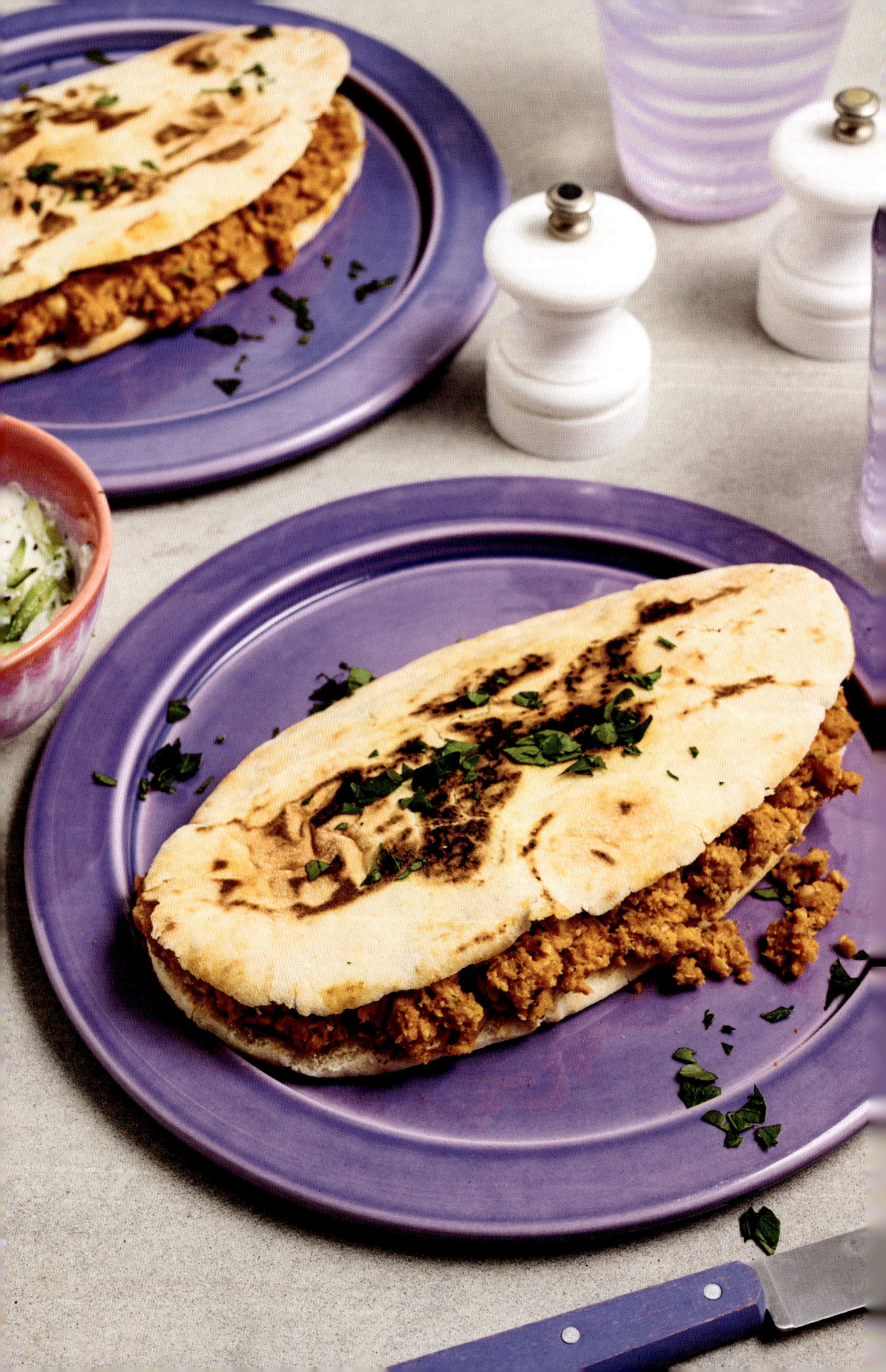

Spicy Chickpea Pitta Breads

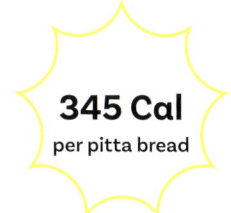
345 Cal per pitta bread

Protein: 15.6g **Fat: 16.4g** **Carbs: 38.9g**

SERVES 2

Crispy on the outside with a warming spiced chickpea filling, these pitta breads are delicious. Pair them with a chopped salad and opt for dipping sauces such as tahini, tzatziki or a garlic herb sauce.

Ingredients

1 × 400g tin of chickpeas, drained
1 small white onion, diced
1 tsp chopped garlic
1 tsp ground cumin
1 tsp ground coriander
½ tsp mild chilli powder
1 tbsp harissa paste
½ tbsp olive oil
3 sprigs of fresh coriander, chopped
2 pitta breads, halved widthways
Salt and pepper
1 sprig of fresh parsley, chopped, to garnish

Method

- Preheat the oven to 220ºC/200ºC fan.
- Next, put the chickpeas into a food processor, along with the onion, garlic, cumin, coriander, chilli powder, harissa paste, olive oil and a pinch of salt and pepper.
- Add the chopped coriander before blitzing for a couple of minutes until it forms a paste.
- Stuff the paste into the pitta breads, before adding to a large dry frying pan. Fry chickpea-side down over a medium heat for a minute before toasting the other sides for 30 seconds each.
- Transfer to a baking tray and cook for 10 minutes. Remove and garnish with fresh parsley.

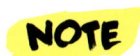

These will last in the fridge for 2–3 days.

Sweet Chilli Halloumi Salad

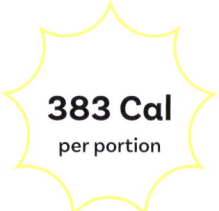

383 Cal per portion

Protein: 32.5g **Fat: 20.4g** **Carbs: 16.1g**

SERVES 2

I don't know about you but my salads have to have some flavour otherwise I'm not interested! The star of this recipe are the bites of halloumi that are seasoned in garlic and paprika before being tossed with sweet chilli for an eye-watering bite every time. Customise with your favourite salad items if you wish (I also like to add crispy onions or pomegranate seeds from time to time), before drizzling with the garlic herb yoghurt drizzle.

Ingredients

225g reduced-fat halloumi, cut into cubes and patted dry

1 tsp garlic granules

½ tsp smoked paprika

35g reduced-sugar sweet chilli sauce

Olive oil spray

100g mixed baby leaf salad

1 small red onion, diced

100g cherry tomatoes, quartered

Garlic herb yoghurt drizzle

50g fat-free Greek yoghurt

½ tsp garlic granules

¼ tsp dried parsley

1 tsp distilled white vinegar

Pinch of salt

Method

- Start by tossing the halloumi in a bowl with the garlic granules, smoked paprika and sweet chilli sauce.
- Next, heat a medium frying pan with a few pumps of olive oil spray. Add the cubed halloumi, ensuring that the pieces are not overlapping. Cook for 4 minutes, turning every 1 minute for even cooking.
- Meanwhile, make the garlic drizzle by mixing together all the ingredients and set to one side.
- Prepare the salad by placing the baby leaf salad in a bowl. Top with the red onion, tomatoes and cooked halloumi bites before drizzling over the garlic herb dressing.

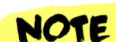

If meal prepping this recipe, ensure that the sauce is stored separately and drizzle it over before eating. This recipe should last for up to 2 days in an airtight container in the fridge.

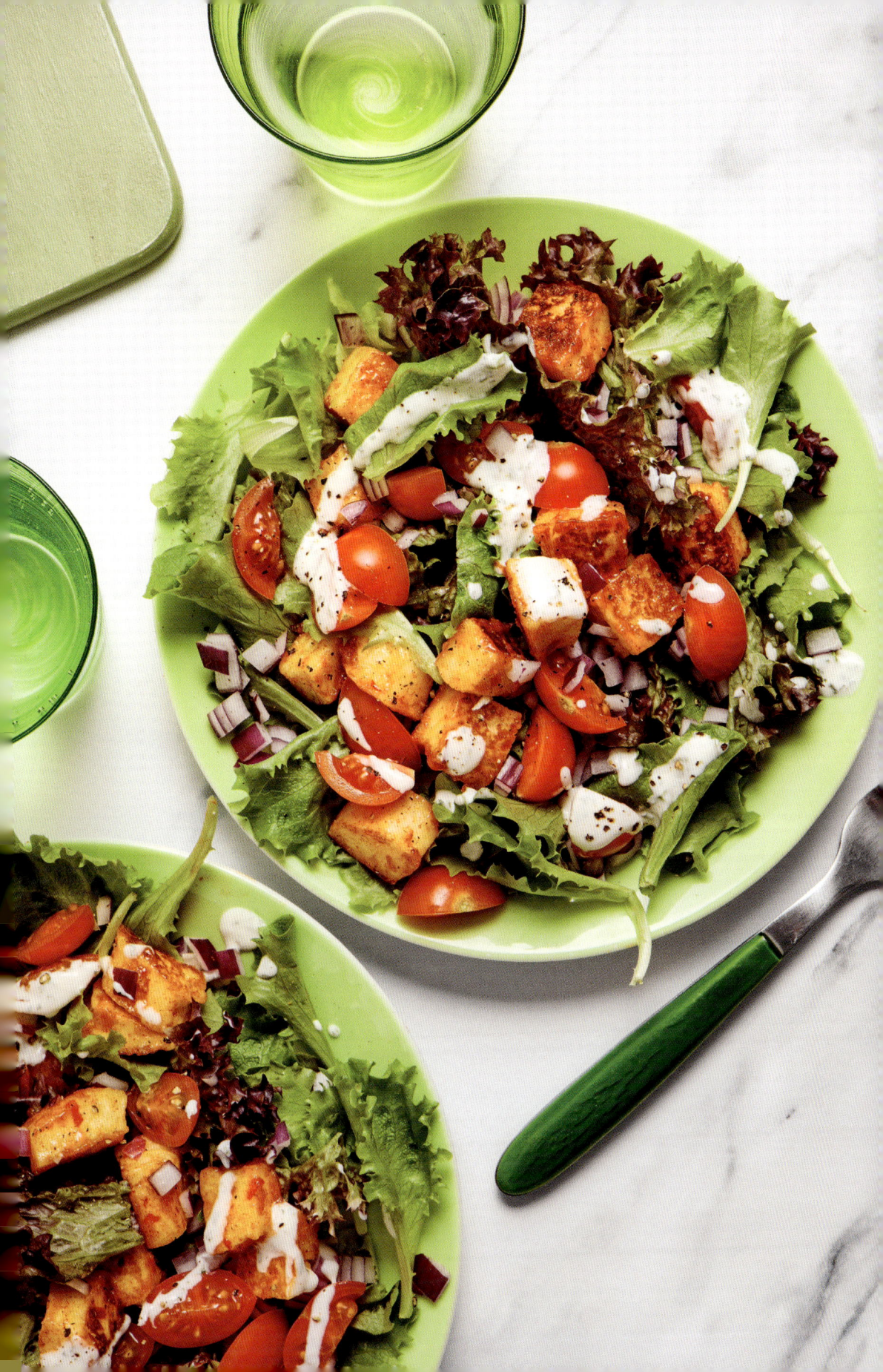

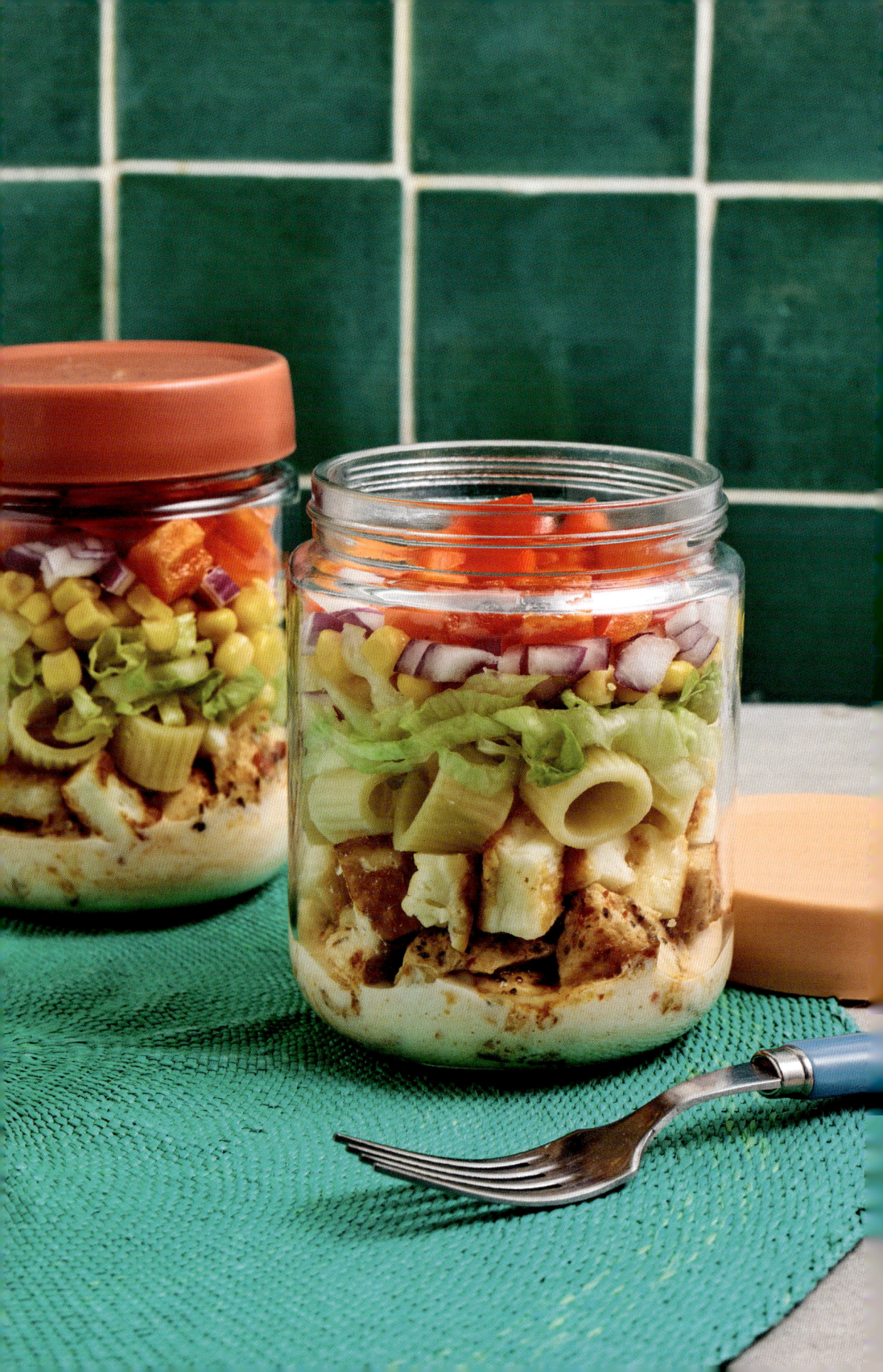

Peri Chicken Pasta Salad Jars

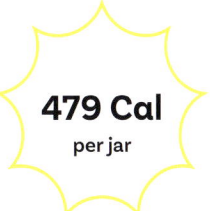

479 Cal per jar

Protein: 45.3g Fat: 8.7g Carbs: 47.3g

SERVES 2

Say goodbye to soggy salads on the go with these pasta salad jars. By layering the salad with the sauce at the bottom so that it comes up as far as the lettuce everything stays nice and crispy. This flavour combination is truly my favourite, it has peri chicken, halloumi and pasta – lots of nutrients in your salad plus a delicious homemade peri dressing.

Ingredients

100g dried pasta (I use rigatoni)
Olive oil spray
50g reduced-fat halloumi, diced
200g skinless chicken breast, cut into 2.5cm cubes
1 tsp peri seasoning
1 red pepper, diced
1 red onion, diced
40g sweetcorn
½ × 130g bag of shredded lettuce

Peri sauce
80g fat-free Greek yoghurt
10g lighter than light mayonnaise
1 tbsp peri sauce
½ tsp garlic granules
Pinch of salt

Method

- Start by putting the pasta into a large pan of salted boiling water. Cook according to the packet instructions.
- Heat a large frying pan over a high heat. Spray with a few pumps of olive oil, add the diced halloumi and cook for 3–4 minutes, until golden.
- While the halloumi cooks, season the chicken with the peri seasoning. Rub in thoroughly and set to one side.
- Once the halloumi is cooked, remove from the pan. Add the chicken to the same pan and cook over a medium-high heat for 8–9 minutes or until cooked through. Remove from the heat and leave to cool slightly.
- While the chicken cooks, mix the sauce ingredients in a bowl.
- Once the pasta is cooked, drain and rinse under cold water to help the cooling process.
- When all the food is ready, start layering the pasta salad in a jar (I find a Mason jar around 500–750ml works best). Start with the peri sauce, then add the chicken, halloumi, cooked pasta, red pepper, red onion and sweetcorn and finish with the shredded lettuce.

NOTE

The longer you leave the chicken to cool, the better. The jars will keep in the fridge for a day with the lettuce added, or up to 3–4 days without the lettuce, which you can either add fresh or sub for spinach.

Chicken Caesar Salad Pitta Breads

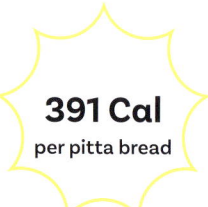

391 Cal per pitta bread

| Protein: 37.8g | Fat: 8.4g | Carbs: 35.4g |

SERVES 2

 AF

I think we can all agree, chicken Caesar salads are elite. Here, some of the bacon is stirred into the homemade Caesar sauce along with the Parmesan for an addictive combination. This is then stuffed into pitta breads, with romaine lettuce and shredded chicken breast. If you fancy added crunch, you can top the pittas with crispy bacon bits or crispy onions, found near the salad toppers in supermarkets.

Ingredients

150g skinless chicken breast, flattened slightly

3 bacon medallions

15g Parmesan, grated

2 soft white pitta breads (I use Warburtons), sliced

¾ romaine lettuce chopped

Salt and pepper

½ tsp dried chives, to garnish

Caesar sauce

70g fat-free Greek yoghurt

10g lighter than light mayonnaise

¼ tbsp Worcestershire sauce

1 tsp lemon juice

¼ tsp garlic granules

¼ tsp Dijon mustard

Method

- Start by preheating the oven to 220ºC/200ºC fan.
- While the oven heats, add the chicken to a baking tray and season with salt and pepper. Place in the oven for 10-12 minutes, until cooked through.
- Next, preheat the grill to medium-high. Once hot, put the bacon medallions under it and grill for 4-6 minutes, turning partway through, until cooked.
- While the bacon cooks, make the Caesar sauce by combining all the ingredients with salt and pepper to taste.
- Once combined, stir through the grated Parmesan.
- Next, toast the pitta breads.
- Stuff the pitta breads with the lettuce. Shred the cooked chicken using two forks and add it to the pittas.
- Cut the bacon into small square shapes. Stir half into the Caesar sauce and pour the sauce into the pitta bread. Finish by scattering with the remaining bacon on top, followed by the dried chives.

Air fryer Cook the chicken at 190ºC for 8-10 minutes, turning partway through. The bacon can be cooked at 190ºC for 4-6 minutes.

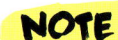

The pitta breads will keep for up to 2 days in the fridge before the lettuce starts to deteriorate. The filling can be kept in the fridge for up to 4 days in an airtight container.

Naked Chicken Kebab

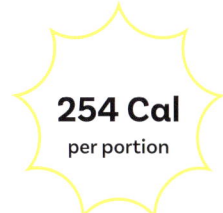

254 Cal per portion

| Protein: 40.4g | Fat: 4.3g | Carbs: 11.5g |

SERVES 2

All the yummy flavours of a kebab turned into a salad for a lighter lunch. If you do have more time on your hands, you can marinate the chicken for anywhere from 10 minutes to a few hours to allow the flavours to deepen. And if you fancy some carbs with this lunch, the filling is banging in a soft pitta bread.

Ingredients

250g skinless chicken breast, cut into 2.5cm cubes

30g fat-free natural yoghurt

1 tsp oregano

¾ tsp cumin

1 tsp smoked paprika

1 tbsp lemon juice

1 tbsp tomato purée

120g mixed leaves

½ cucumber, cut into small dice

2 salad tomatoes, cut into small dice

1 small red onion, diced

1 tbsp chilli sauce

Salt and pepper

Garlic yoghurt sauce

50g fat-free natural yoghurt

½ tsp garlic granules

½ tsp parsley

1 tsp distilled white vinegar

Method

- Start by putting the diced chicken into a bowl. Next, add the yoghurt, oregano, cumin, smoked paprika and a pinch of salt and pepper. Pour in the lemon juice and add the tomato purée. Mix well to combine.
- Next, heat a large frying pan over a medium-high heat.
- Add the chicken to the pan and fry for 8 minutes, until the chicken is cooked through.
- While the chicken cooks, make the yoghurt sauce by mixing all the ingredients with a pinch of salt and pepper and set to one side.
- Once the chicken is cooked, put the salad leaves into a bowl. Top with the cooked chicken, and put the diced vegetables on the side. Drizzle over the garlic yoghurt sauce along with the chilli sauce.

Air fryer Thread the chicken onto metal skewers. If you have wooden ones, make sure you soak them for 30 minutes prior to cooking. Air fry for 16 minutes at 200°C.

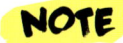

To take this for lunch on the go, I recommend storing the sauce in a separate pot to help keep the salad fresh.

BLT Bagels

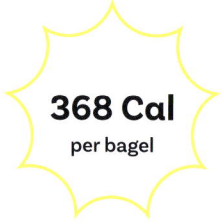

368 Cal per bagel

Protein: 20g   **Fat: 6g**   **Carbs: 49.9g**

SERVES 2

Nothing quite beats the freshness of a BLT for me, especially teamed with a creamy sauce laced with tomato, garlic and Parmesan and served on a bagel. I tend to keep a batch of the filling in the fridge; that way I always have something prepared for those days when I'm starving and ready to devour my whole kitchen.

Ingredients

6 bacon medallions
20g lighter than light mayonnaise
50g fat-free Greek yoghurt
¼ tsp garlic granules
5g Parmesan, grated
2 salad tomatoes, diced
2 bagels, sliced in half through the middle
1 little gem lettuce, chopped
Salt and pepper

Method

- Start by preheating the grill to medium-high.
- Put the bacon medallions under the grill and cook for 4-6 minutes, turning partway through, until cooked through.
- While the bacon cooks, mix together the mayo, yoghurt and garlic granules with a generous amount of black pepper and salt to taste. Once combined, stir through the grated Parmesan and the salad tomatoes. Set to one side.
- Place the bagels in a toaster for a couple of minutes until lightly golden.
- Once the bacon is cooked, slice into small strips and fold into the mayonnaise mixture.
- Top each half of the bagel with lettuce followed by the creamy bacon mixture.

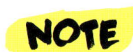

You can prep this filling and keep it in the fridge for up to 3 days.

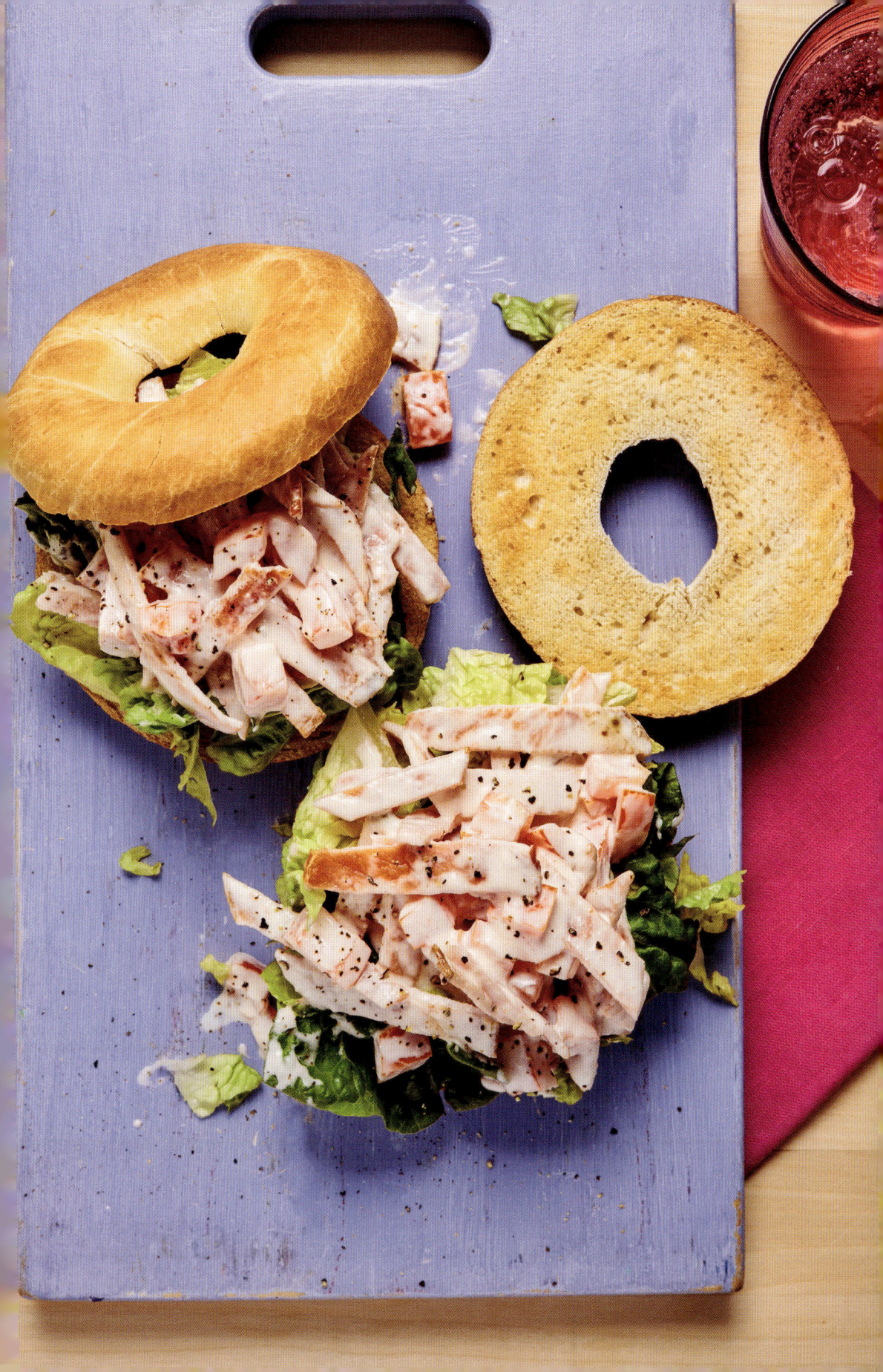

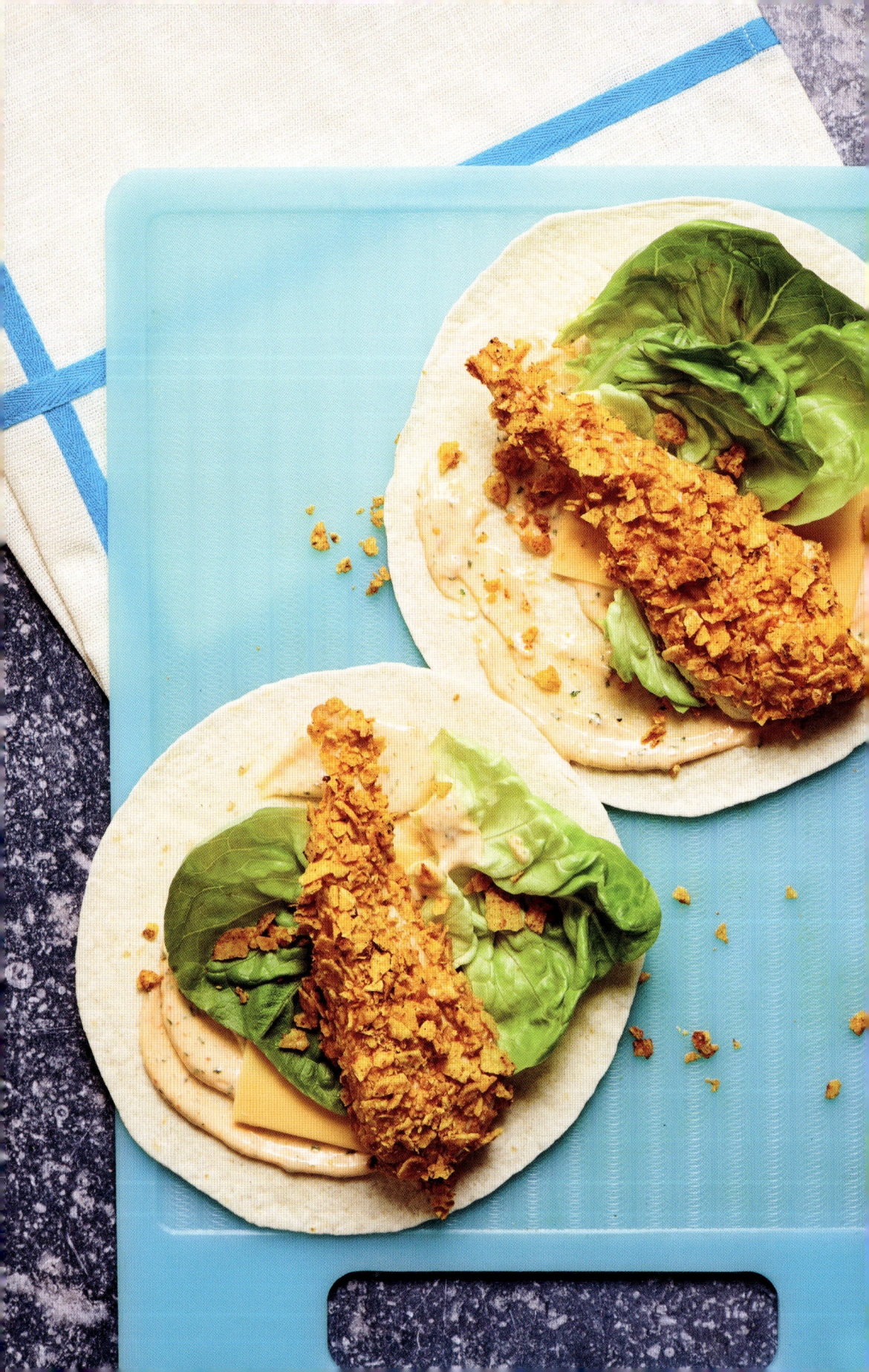

Crispy Chicken Snack Wraps

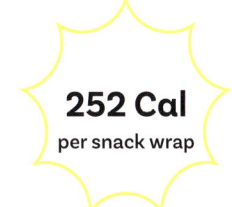

252 Cal per snack wrap

Protein: 23.1g   **Fat: 7g**   **Carbs: 19.1g**

MAKES 2

AF

When a certain fast food chain stopped snack wraps, that meant rustling them up at home, and I'm not mad about it. My version is less processed and has more protein to help keep you fuller than the wraps otherwise would. This combination uses chilli heatwave tortilla chips to coat the chicken with a seasoned spicy-style mayo sauce.

Ingredients

1 tsp garlic granules
1 tsp onion granules
1 tsp smoked paprika
2 × 60g chicken breast tenders
15g chilli tortilla chips, finely crushed
20g egg whites
2 mini tortilla wraps
4 roundhead lettuce leaves
1 light cheese slice, halved

Sauce

30g lighter than light mayonnaise
½ tsp sriracha sauce
1 tsp distilled white vinegar
¼ tsp dried parsley

Method

- Preheat the oven to 205°C/185°C fan.
- Start by mixing the garlic and onion granules and smoked paprika together in a bowl to make a seasoning.
- Set aside ¼ teaspoon of the seasoning for the sauce. Spilt the remaining amount in half, and use half to coat the chicken on both sides, and half to season the tortilla chips, mixing well.
- Dip each tender into the egg white, shaking off the excess egg, and then dip into the crushed tortilla chips.
- Transfer to a non-stick baking tray (or line a tray with baking paper) and bake in the oven for 18 minutes.
- While the chicken cooks, mix together all the sauce ingredients with the ¼ teaspoon of reserved seasoning. Add a tablespoon of hot water if needed to get your desired consistency.
- Warm the tortilla wraps in the microwave on high for 10 seconds.
- On each wrap, layer the sauce, followed by the lettuce, cheese slice and cooked chicken, leave some space at the bottom. Fold up the bottom first, followed by the two sides and wrap each in foil or parchment paper to hold it together.

Air fryer Cook the chicken at 185°C for 14 minutes.

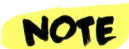

If wrapping these up for later, allow to cool completely. I would only keep them in the fridge for one day.

Chicken Mushroom 'Pot Noodle'

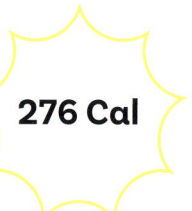

276 Cal

Protein: 19.8g   **Fat: 3.3g**   **Carbs: 39.5g**

SERVES 1

Oh, how a Pot Noodle takes me back to my student days. They are still something I crave at lunchtime. Here I've made a healthier, more nutritious and filling version of the nation's favourite, which requires little prep and you can take to work.

Ingredients

Olive oil spray

40g baby mushrooms, diced

25g sweetcorn

50g fine egg noodles

3 tsp light soy sauce

50g cooked skinless chicken breast, diced

Spice mix

1 chicken stock cube, crumbled

½ tsp garlic granules

½ tsp onion granules

¼ tsp ground ginger

¼ tsp dried chives

⅛ tsp dried sage

To serve

225ml boiling water

Method

- Heat a frying pan over a medium-high heat, spray with olive oil spray and pan-fry the mushrooms for a couple of minutes. Once they are soft and starting to brown, add the sweetcorn for a minute, then remove from the heat.

- While the mushrooms cook, parboil the noodles for half the recommended time on the packet in a large pan of water. Once the time is up, drain and rinse under cold water.

- While the food cools, mix together all of the spice mix ingredients in a bowl.

- To a heatproof jar or glass container, add the spice mix followed by the soy sauce. Top with the mushroom and sweetcorn mix, followed by the diced cooked chicken and noodles.

- Cover and keep in the fridge for up to 4 days. When ready to reheat, leave the jars at room temperature for 20–30 minutes before pouring over 225ml of boiling water. Give it all a good stir before covering and leaving to stand for a few minutes.

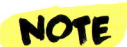

I like to slice up some spring onion and put it in a separate bag when on the go, to add as a garnish.

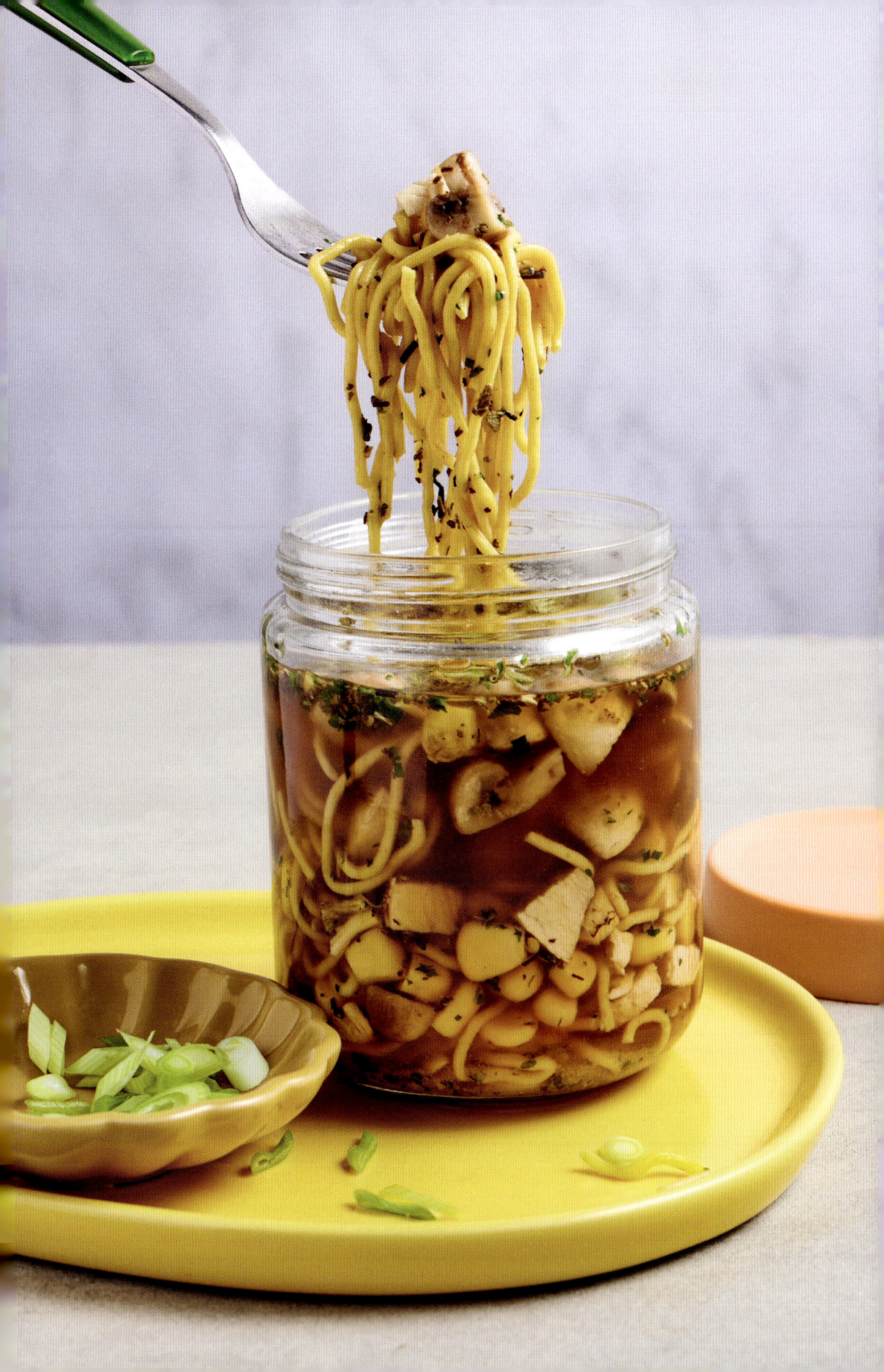

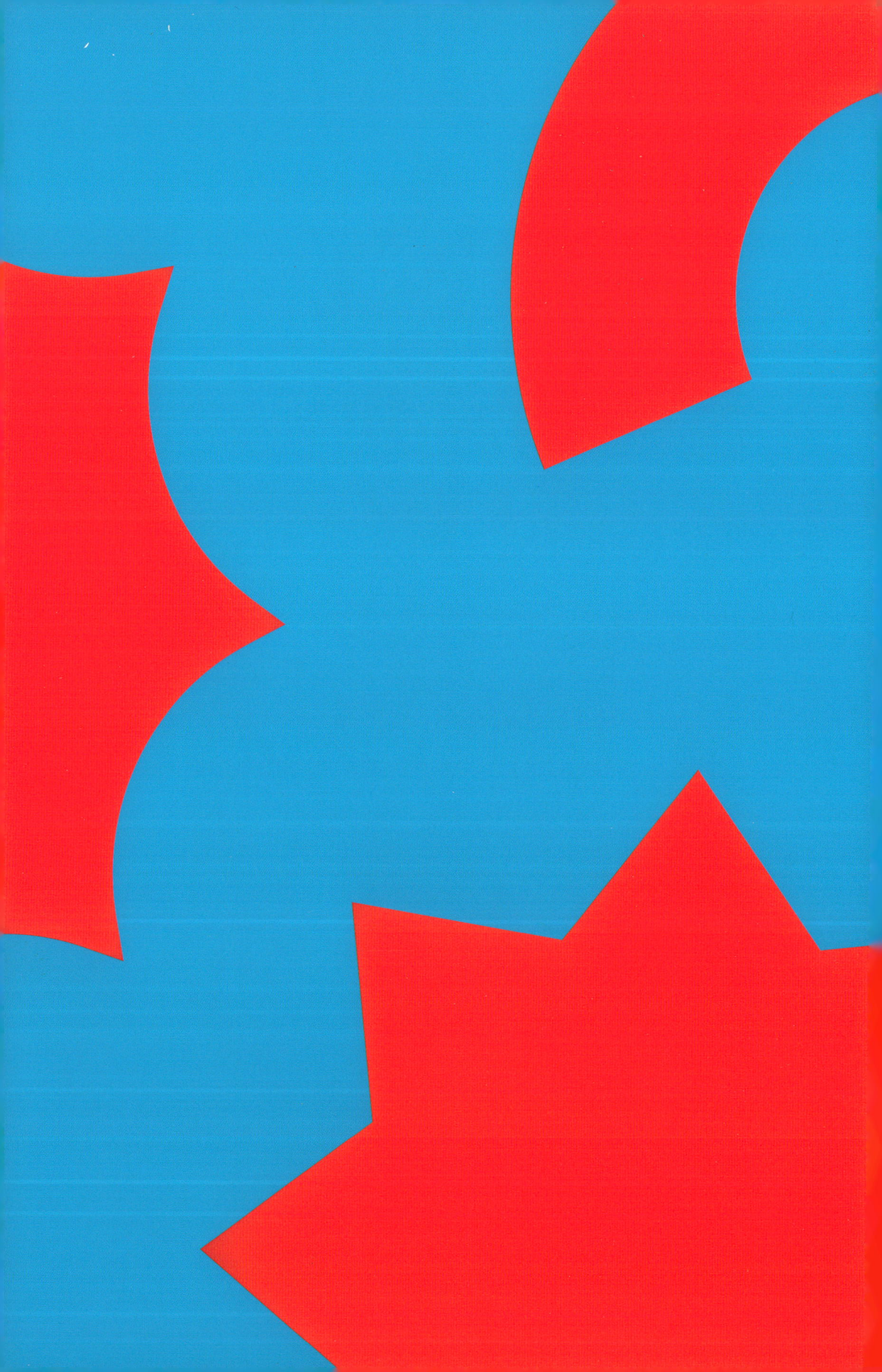

Three

LIGHT
LUNCHES

Crispy Beef Quesadillas

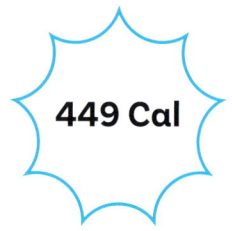
449 Cal

Protein: 40.7g **Fat: 14.2g** **Carbs: 37.6g**

SERVES 1

Quesadillas are one of my go-tos for a speedy lunch option. These are crispy on the outside and stuffed full of a tomato taco beef mix with oozy melted mozzarella. I like to serve them with a side salad topped with a dollop of Greek yoghurt or ranch dressing.

Ingredients

Olive oil spray
100g lean beef mince
½ small white onion, diced
1 tbsp taco seasoning
½ tsp chopped garlic
1 tsp tomato purée
1 tbsp tomato salsa
50ml water
1 tortilla wrap
30g mozzarella, grated
A sprig of fresh coriander, chopped, to garnish

Method

- Start by spraying a frying pan with olive oil spray and placing it on a medium-high heat. Add the beef mince, along with the onion, and use a wooden spoon to break down the mince into smaller pieces.

- Fry for a few minutes, then add the taco seasoning, garlic, tomato purée, salsa and water. Mix well to combine for a further minute or until the liquid has thickened.

- Put the tortilla wrap into a clean separate pan with no oil on a medium heat. On one half, spread out the mozzarella, top with the beef mix and fold the other half of the wrap over the top. Leave for 2 minutes before flipping for a further minute, until the outside of the quesadilla is toasted and the cheese has melted.

- Remove from the heat and cut the quesadilla into four triangles. Sprinkle over the chopped coriander.

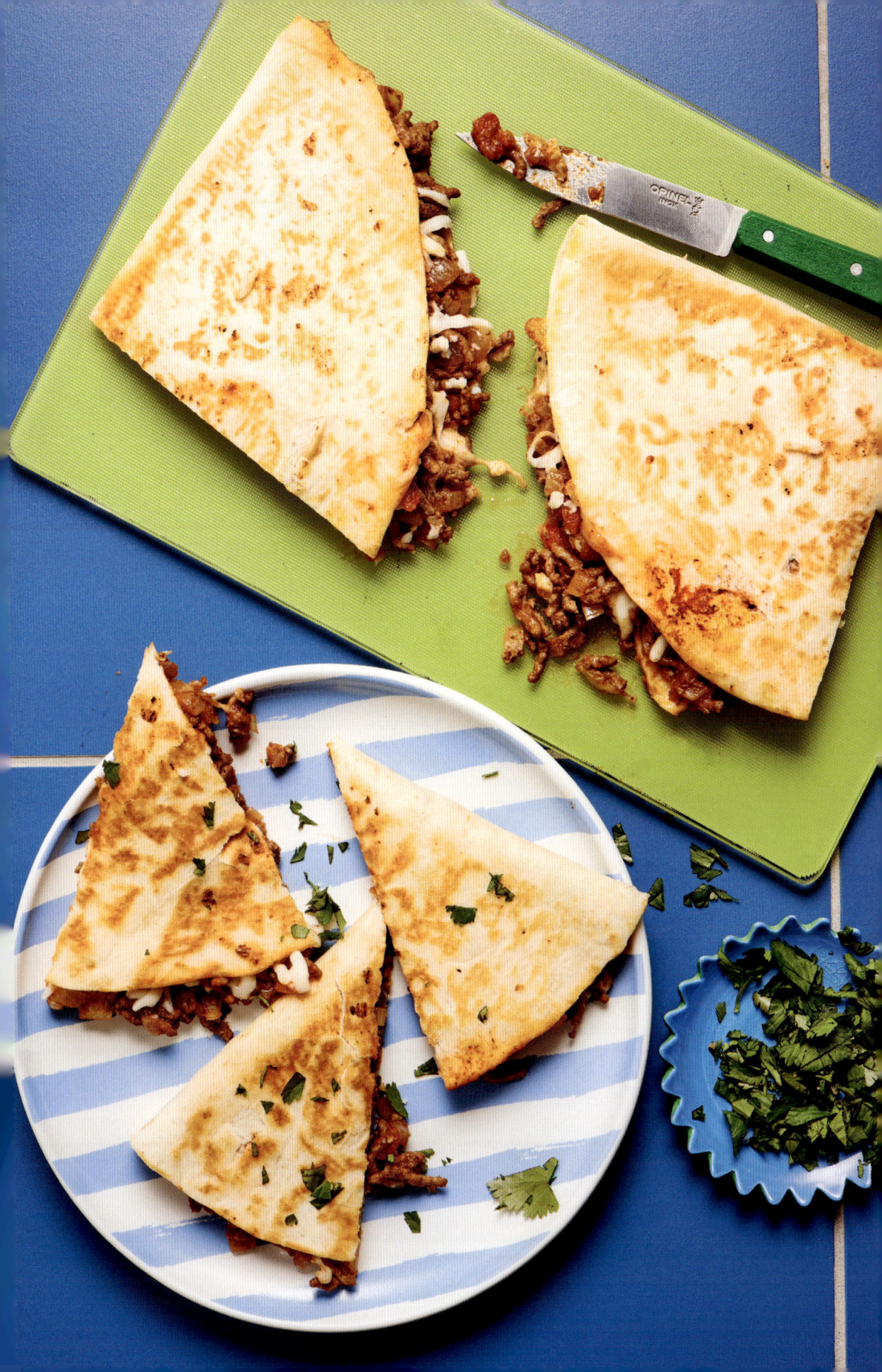

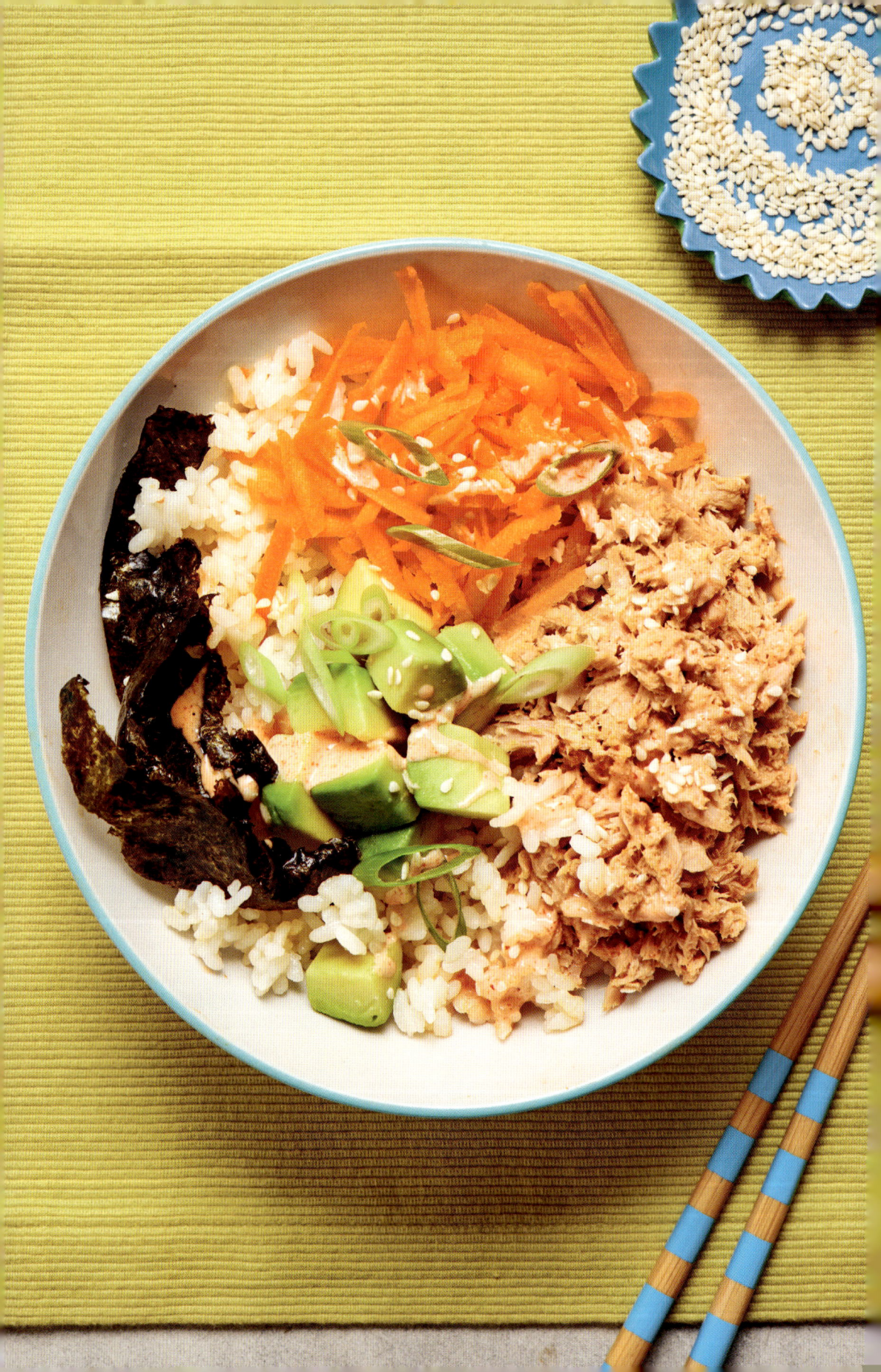

Spicy Tuna Sushi Bowls

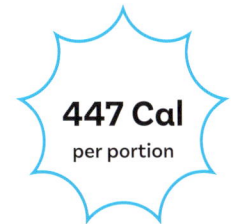

447 Cal per portion

Protein: 30.1g **Fat: 14.4g** **Carbs: 49.2g**

SERVES 2

If, like me, you're forever craving sushi but can't be bothered to make it, opt for these super-quick sushi-style bowls instead. Anti-tuna fans, don't fret – simply swap the tuna for canned salmon or shredded chicken. Other veggies, such as edamame beans and cucumber also go well in this bowl. If you can't get your hands on Kewpie mayo, just swap it for normal mayonnaise, and any white rice will do.

Ingredients

2 × 145g tins of tuna in brine, drained (drained weight 102g each)

1½ tbsp sriracha sauce

20g Kewpie mayo

1 × 250g packet of microwave sticky rice

2 tbsp light soy sauce

2 small carrots, grated

60g avocado, diced

2 sheets of sushi nori (seaweed)

1 spring onion, sliced

1 tsp sesame seeds

Method

- Put both cans of drained tuna into a mixing bowl. Add 1 tablespoon of the sriracha sauce, followed by the Kewpie mayo. Use a fork to combine the sauces well with the tuna and set to one side.

- Next, microwave the rice as per the packet instructions.

- Divide the rice between two bowls, drizzling the soy sauce over each, before adding the grated carrots and diced avocado. Tear the pieces of sushi nori into strips and add to the bowl. Drizzle over the remaining sriracha sauce and garnish with the spring onion and sesame seeds.

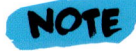

You can prep these bowls ahead of time. Most sushi is consumed cold so these are a perfect on-the-go lunch. Ensure the filling is completely cool before storing in an airtight container for up to 2 days. I recommend adding the avocado fresh at the time of eating so that it doesn't brown.

Speedy Tomato Soup

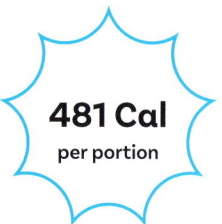

Protein: 36.8g **Fat: 15.5g** **Carbs: 99.4g**

SERVES 2

This speedy soup is made with mostly pantry ingredients. For extra comfort, it's paired with a golden cheese toastie for dipping. I like to add a dash of cream to my tomato soup, but this tastes just as delicious without if you don't have any in your fridge. Switch things up by adding a teaspoon of pesto or harissa when simmering to incorporate different flavours.

Ingredients

1 white onion, diced
1 tsp chopped garlic
1 × 400g tin good-quality chopped tomatoes
1 tbsp tomato purée
100ml hot vegetable stock
½ tsp Italian herb seasoning
1 tsp granulated sweetener (optional)
10g light butter
4 slices of sourdough bread (45g each)
4 mozzarella slices (the thin slices from a packet)
10g single cream

Method

- Add the onion and garlic to a saucepan. Sweat for 2 minutes before adding in the chopped tomatoes, tomato purée, vegetable stock, herb seasoning and sweetener, if using. Turn down to a medium heat and simmer, covered, for 8 minutes.
- Meanwhile, thinly spread the butter on one side of each slice of bread. It's just enough to encourage browning. Place two slices of the bread, butter-side down, in a large frying pan over a medium heat. Top with the mozzarella slices and remaining slices of bread, butter-side up.
- After 2 minutes flip the toastie and repeat for the same amount of time with the pan covered to encourage the cheese to melt, keeping an eye on it to make sure it doesn't burn.
- Once the 8 minutes of simmering time is up, transfer the tomato mix to a food processor or blender, or use an immersion blender. Blend to a smooth soup, then return to the pan and add the cream.
- Serve the soup with the cheese toastie.

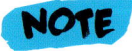

You can meal prep this soup ahead of time and easily double up the ingredients to create a larger batch. Ensure that you store in an airtight container and that the soup is cool prior to refrigerating for up to 3 days.

Spicy Chicken Pizza Wrap

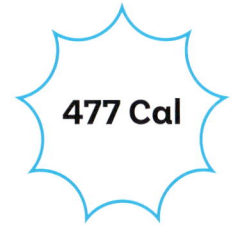

| Protein: 40.5g | Fat: 16g | Carbs: 40.1g |

SERVES 1

One of my favourite go-to lunches is a pizza wrap. It hits those cravings you may have for pizza but keeps things fresh and light. I love pairing mine with a nice crisp salad to feel really satisfied. The possibilities for this wrap are endless, but this variation uses fajita seasoning and chipotle paste to give it that spicy flavour. You can swap the chicken breast for lean beef mince if you fancy a change.

Ingredients

100g skinless chicken breast, cut into 2.5cm cubes
1 tsp fajita seasoning
1 tsp chipotle paste
Olive oil spray
1 tortilla wrap
45g pizza sauce
¼ red onion, diced
25g mozzarella, grated
15g peri mayonnaise
1 sprig of fresh coriander, chopped
3 jalapeños

Method

- In a bowl, season the chicken breast with the fajita seasoning, chipotle paste and olive oil spray and air fry for 8 minutes at 190°C. Alternatively, pan fry the seasoned chicken in olive oil spray until cooked through.

- Grab your tortilla wrap. Spread the pizza sauce over it before topping with the chicken, onion and mozzarella. Spray a few squirts of olive oil around the edges and brush for a golden crispy edge.

- Place in the air fryer for 5 minutes at 190°C. Alternatively, bake in the oven on a non-stick baking tray at 210°C/190°C fan for 8-10 minutes.

- Carefully remove the wrap from the air fryer. Drizzle over the peri mayonnaise and sprinkle over the coriander and jalapeños.

Buffalo Chicken Lettuce Wraps

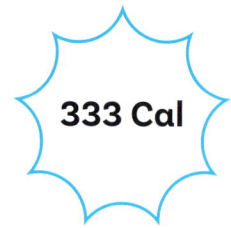

333 Cal

Protein: 42.4g   Fat: 14.4g   Carbs: 7.2g

SERVES 1

For the days you need a lighter lunch, opt for these buffalo chicken lettuce wraps. Lettuce leaves are stuffed with saucy buffalo chicken pieces with crunchy celery, grated cheddar and spring onion and a cooling yoghurt ranch dressing. You can easily switch out the celery for diced tomato and red onion and use blue cheese dressing for some variety. My top tip for making creamy sauces go further and to use fewer calories is to always mix them with some Greek yoghurt!

Ingredients

130g skinless chicken breast, cut into 2.5cm cubes
½ tsp smoked paprika
½ tsp onion granules
½ tsp garlic granules
Olive oil spray
10g ranch dressing
20g fat-free Greek yoghurt
5g light butter
15ml buffalo sauce
4 large butterhead or romaine lettuce leaves
1½ small celery sticks, finely chopped
10g Red Leicester or reduced-fat cheddar, grated
1 spring onion, finely diced
Salt and pepper

Method

- Start by seasoning the chicken with the smoked paprika, onion granules, garlic granules and some salt and pepper.
- Spray a frying pan with a few pumps of olive oil spray. Add the chicken to the pan and cook over a high heat for 5 minutes.
- Once the chicken has cooked, add the butter and toss to cover the chicken. Add the buffalo sauce to cover the chicken and remove from the heat.
- Meanwhile, in a bowl, mix together the ranch dressing and yoghurt until well combined, then set to one side.
- Double up the lettuce leaves, then top with the cooked chicken and chopped celery. Drizzle over the yoghurt ranch sauce, then add the grated cheese and garnish with the spring onion.

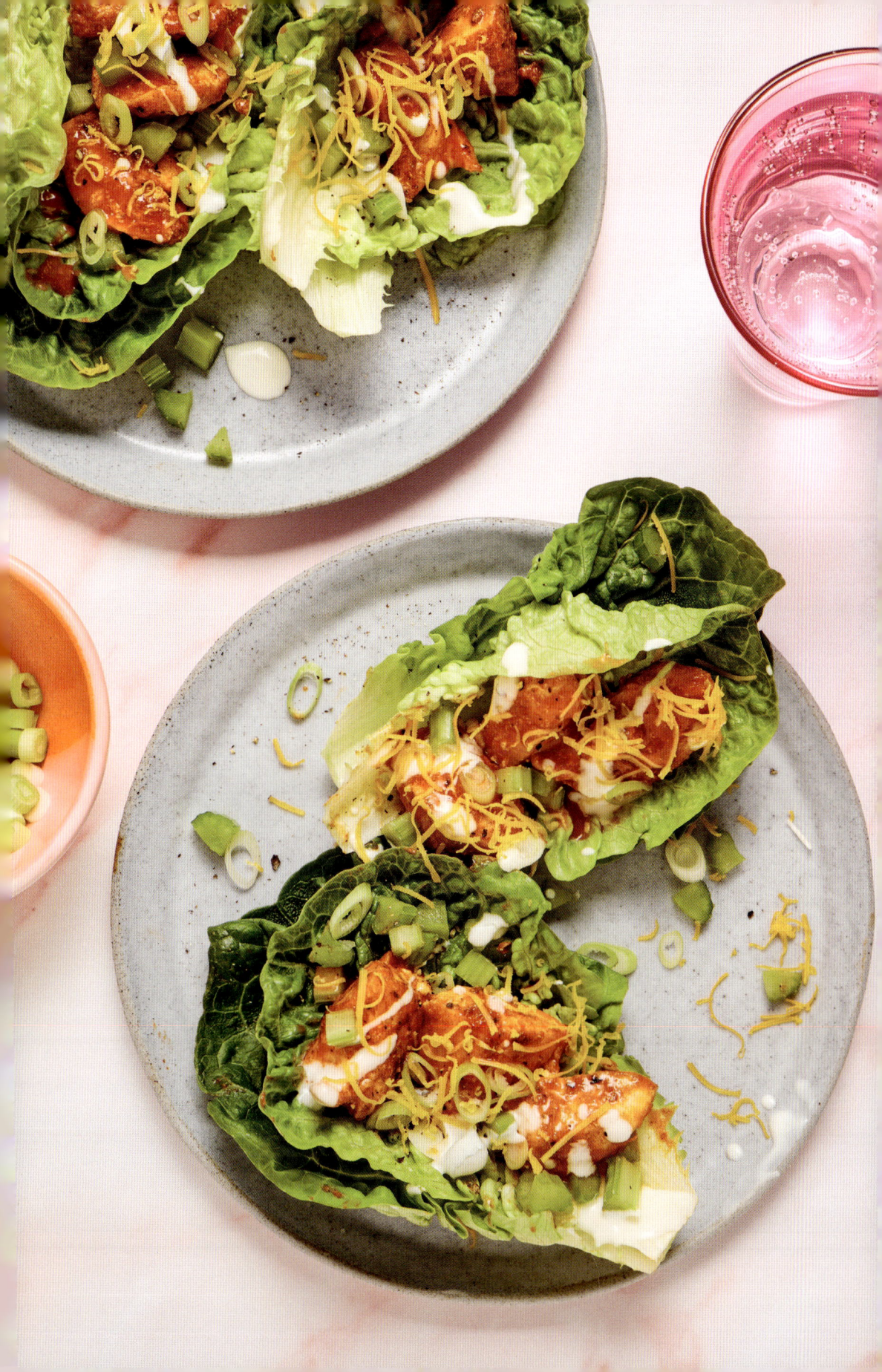

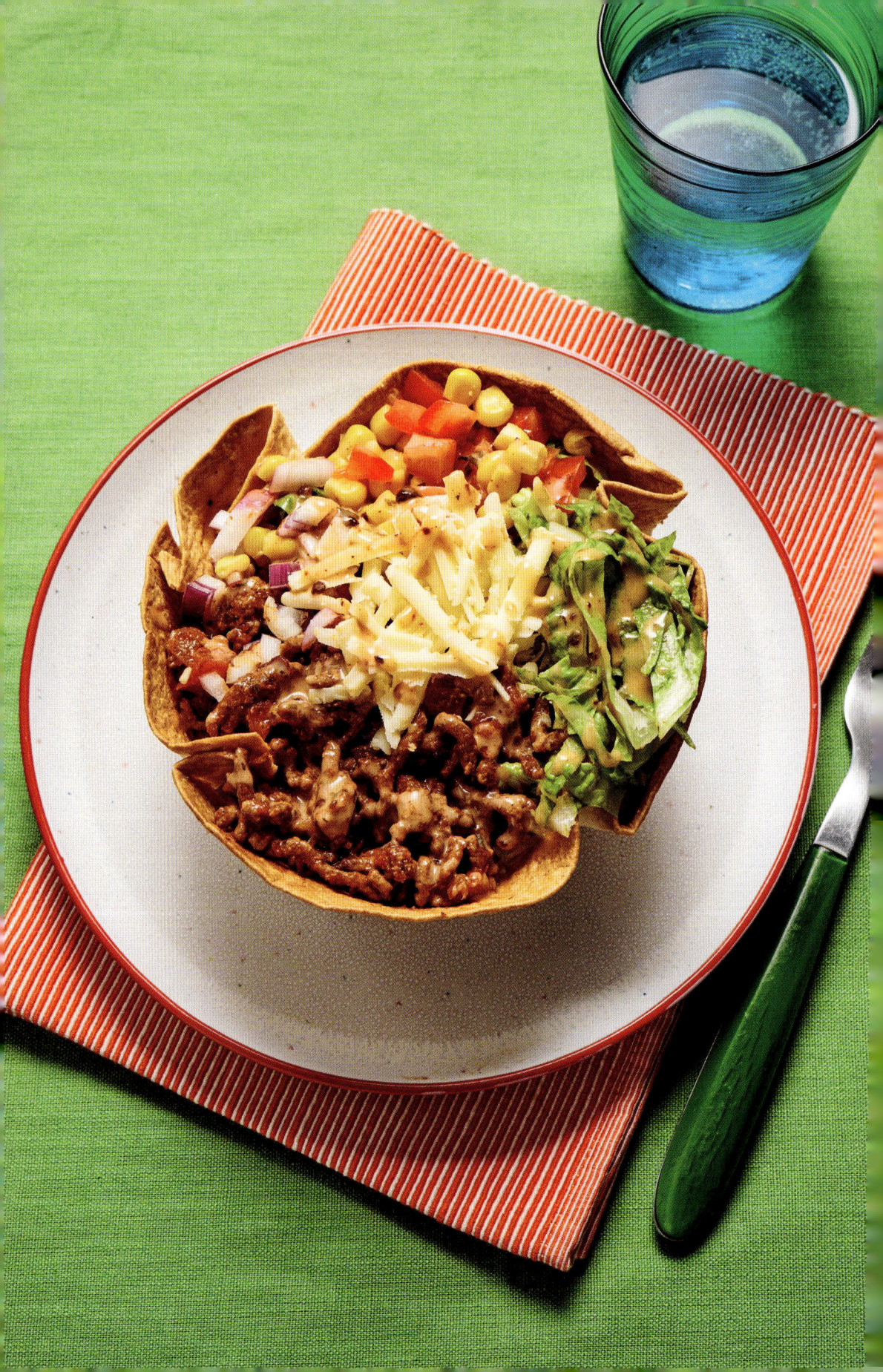

Taco Beef Crispy Basket Bowl

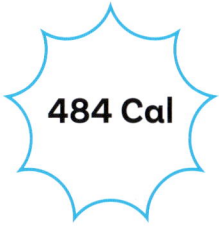

484 Cal

Protein: 37.4g **Fat: 15g** **Carbs: 43.4g**

SERVES 1

Crispy tortilla bowls are so easy to make and a fun way to eat your taco salad. Piled high with salad for nourishment, mouthwatering taco beef, a chipotle ranch drizzle and cheddar for tastebud heaven. Use this recipe without the tortilla bowl for a lighter lunch on the go.

Ingredients

1 tortilla wrap
olive oil spray
100g lean beef mince
1 tbsp taco seasoning
50ml water
30g salsa
¼ tsp chipotle paste
10g ranch dressing
2 handfuls of shredded lettuce
1 salad tomato, diced
½ small red onion, diced
20g sweetcorn
10g reduced-fat cheddar, grated
1 sprig of fresh coriander, chopped

Method

- Preheat the oven to 220°C/200°C fan.
- Grab a small ovenproof bowl and place the tortilla inside. Push in gently until the whole wrap is inside the bowl, creating a bowl shape itself. Place on top of a baking tray and pop in the oven for 7 minutes.
- Meanwhile, spray a frying pan with a few pumps of olive oil spray. Add the beef mince and fry for 4-5 minutes, until browned.
- Once the beef is brown, add the taco seasoning, water and salsa. Cook for 2 minutes, until there's virtually no sauce left.
- While the sauce thickens, mix together the chipotle paste and ranch sauce. If needed, loosen with a teaspoon of water to get your desired consistency.
- When the beef is ready, grab the cooked tortilla bowl. Load firstly with the shredded lettuce, then the cooked taco beef, followed by the tomato, red onion, sweetcorn and cheese. Drizzle over the chipotle ranch sauce and garnish with the fresh coriander.

Ham and Cheese Puff Bakes

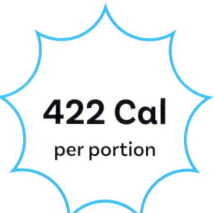

422 Cal per portion

| Protein: 22.2g | Fat: 18.9g | Carbs: 30.9g |

MAKES 2

 AF

For the moments where you're craving golden flaky pastry, this simple recipe is all you need. My favourite part about this recipe is using cheese triangles to spread over one side of the puff pastry. It melts down when baking, almost becoming a cheese sauce, which makes it feel a little cheekier than it is.

Ingredients

150g reduced-fat pre-rolled puff pastry sheet, cut into 2 rectangles

2 lightest cheese triangles (I use Laughing Cow)

100g thick-cut cooked ham, cut into small pieces

30g reduced-fat cheddar

1 medium egg, whisked

90g baby leaf salad

70g cherry tomatoes, quartered

15ml balsamic glaze

Method

- Preheat the oven to 220°C/200°C fan.
- Next, place the puff pastry rectangles on a piece of baking paper and roll out slightly using a rolling pin, then transfer the paper and rectangles to a baking tray.
- On one half of the rectangle, spread half of the cheese triangle. On the other half put the cut ham and top with the cheddar, ensuring there is a 2.5cm border around the filling.
- Using a pastry brush, brush the egg over the border.
- Next, fold over the pastry from the spread-cheese side towards the ham side. Use a fork to press around the outside edges to seal the pastry. Brush with more egg wash, then score the top a few times to create steam holes.
- Place in the centre of the oven for 15 minutes, until golden.
- While the pastries cook, divide your baby leaf salad between plates. Top with the halved cherry tomatoes and drizzle with the balsamic glaze.
- Remove the pastries and leave to cool slightly before serving.

Air fryer Simply cook the pastries for 10–12 minutes at 180°C.

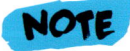

The bakes will keep in the fridge for a few days after cooking – allow to cool completely before storing in the fridge. To reheat, bake in the oven at 220°C/200°C fan for 10 minutes, or heat in the air fryer for 5 minutes at 180°C, until the filling is piping hot.

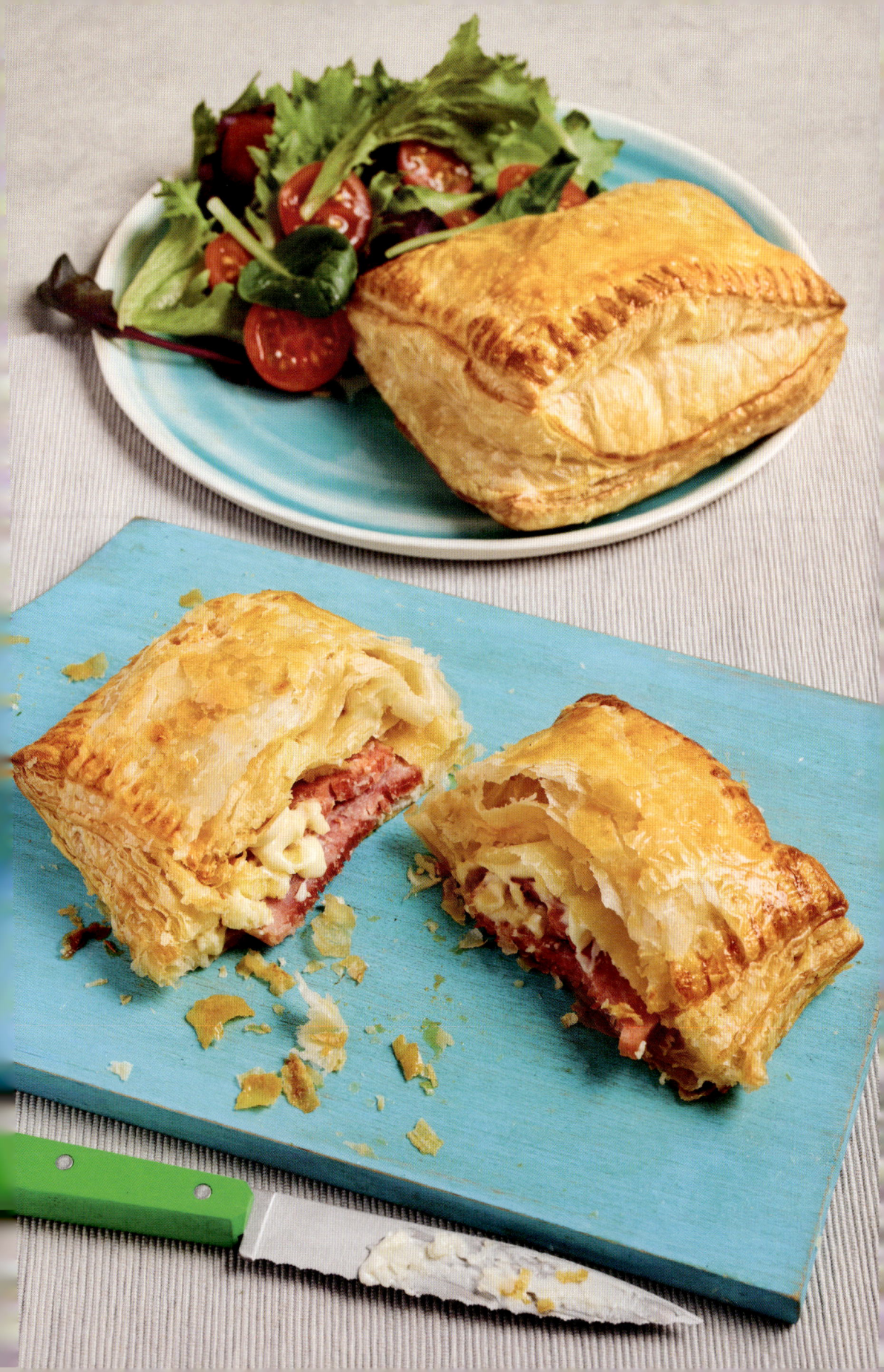

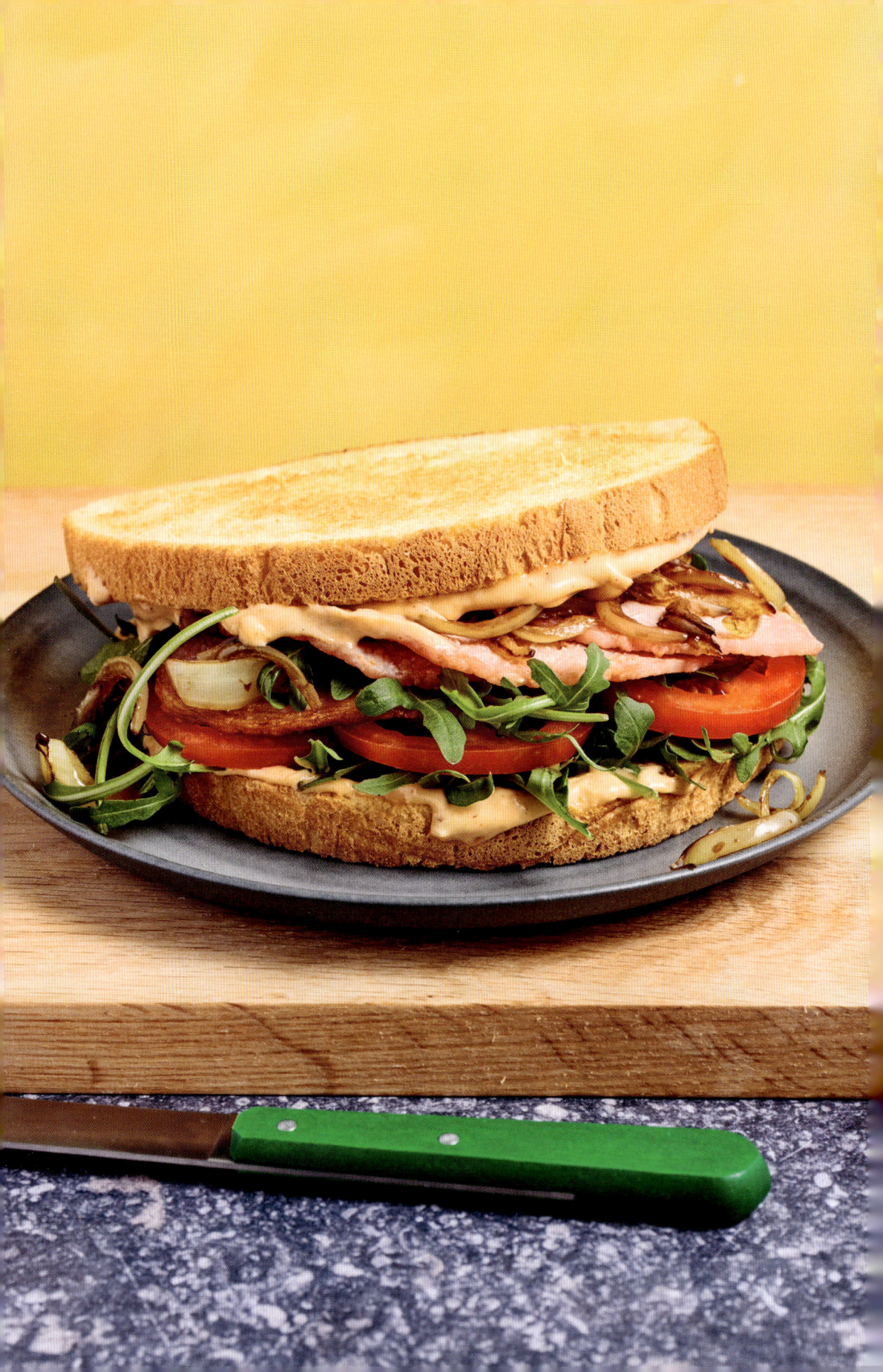

Best Ever Bacon Sandwich

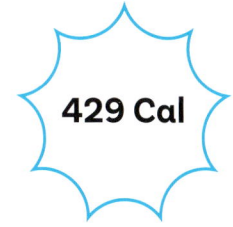
429 Cal

Protein: 23.1g **Fat: 7.7g** **Carbs: 51.4g**

MAKES 1

In my eyes, this really is the best ever bacon sandwich (apart from the classic bacon and ketchup version). Toasted bloomer bread is stacked with rocket, bacon, fried brown onions, thick slices of tomato and a delicious homemade chipotle sauce. It truly is a banger. I sometimes like to add some reduced-fat cheddar or avocado to mix it up, or even throw it on a bake-at-home sourdough baguette.

Ingredients

Olive oil spray

1 small white onion, thinly sliced

4 reduced-fat bacon medallions

1 tsp balsamic glaze

2 slices of white bloomer bread (I use Jacksons; it has 105 calories per slice)

2 handfuls of rocket

1 beef tomato, thinly sliced

Salt and pepper

Chipotle sauce

35g lighter than light mayonnaise (or fat-free Greek yoghurt)

¼ tsp chipotle paste

¼ tsp garlic granules

Pinch of salt

½ tsp distilled white vinegar

Method

- Preheat the grill to medium-high.
- Spray a frying pan with a few pumps of olive oil spray.
- Add the sliced onion to the pan. Fry over a high heat for 8 minutes or so, adding increments of 25ml water to help the browning. Once the onions are brown, turn down the heat.
- Meanwhile, place the bacon under the hot grill. Cook for 7 minutes, turning partway through, until cooked through.
- While the bacon cooks, make the sauce by mixing all the ingredients, then set to one side.
- Add the balsamic glaze to the onions, mix well and turn off the heat.
- Once the bacon is cooked, remove from the grill and set to one side.
- Add the slices of bread to a toaster for a couple of minutes until lightly golden.
- To build the sandwich, place the rocket on a slice of toast, followed by the sliced tomato. Season with salt and pepper before topping with the cooked bacon and onions and the chipotle sauce. Slice and serve.

Pizza-Flavoured Stuffed Peppers

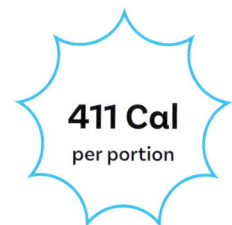

411 Cal
per portion

Protein: 28.9g   Fat: 17.3g   Carbs: 28.2g

SERVES 2

I love pizza, especially the classic pairing of pepperoni and melted cheese. What better way to satisfy a pizza craving than to fuse its flavours with stuffed peppers. You can easily customise these peppers using your favourite pizza toppings.

Ingredients

2 large red peppers, halved, deseeded and membrane removed

Olive oil spray

120g lean beef mince

150g microwave long-grain rice

1 tsp garlic granules

1 tsp dried oregano

1 tsp Italian herb seasoning

1 tbsp tomato purée

150g passata

50g mozzarella, grated

8 pepperoni slices, halved

10g shop-bought garlic herb sauce, to drizzle (optional)

A few basil leaves, chopped (optional)

Method

- Preheat the oven to 220ºC/200ºC fan.
- Put the peppers onto a baking tray. Spray with a few pumps of olive oil spray. Bake for 10 minutes, until slightly softened.
- Meanwhile, heat a large frying pan over a high heat. Spray with a few pumps of olive oil spray, then add the beef mince. Fry for 3-4 minutes, until the beef is almost brown.
- While the beef browns, microwave the rice according to the packet instructions.
- Once the beef is almost brown, add the cooked rice, then turn the heat down to medium before adding the garlic granules, oregano, Italian herb seasoning and tomato purée. Mix to combine, then stir through the passata. Leave over a medium-low heat until the pepper timer is ready.
- Next, equally divide the beef and rice mixture between the peppers.
- Top with the grated mozzarella, followed by the pepperoni slices, then return to the oven for a further 5 minutes to melt the cheese.
- Once cooked, remove from the oven. If you're using them, drizzle over the garlic herb sauce and add the chopped basil.

Air fryer At step 2, place the peppers in the air fryer for 7 minutes at 180ºC. At step 7, place the stuffed peppers in the air fryer for 5 minutes at 180ºC.

Margherita Pesto Flatbread

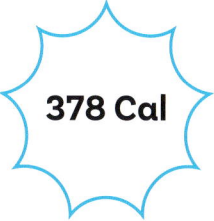

Protein: 21.1g **Fat: 12.3g** **Carbs: 44.6g**

SERVES 1

This is one of my go-to quick lunches. It packs a flavour punch, transports you to summer and leaves you satisfied. I like to have these with a nice salad with balsamic glaze and some cooked chicken when I need an extra protein hit.

Ingredients

1 Greek-style flatbread
Olive oil spray
1 tbsp tomato purée
1 tsp chopped garlic
1 large tomato, thinly sliced
50g reduced-fat mozzarella, sliced
¼ tsp dried oregano
15g reduced-fat green pesto
3 basil leaves, to garnish

Method

- Preheat the oven to 220°C/200°C fan.
- Place the flatbread on a baking tray. Spray lightly with olive oil spray and bake for 4 minutes.
- Remove the flatbread from the oven. Spread over the tomato purée, ensuring the surface of the flatbread is covered. Next, add the chopped garlic on top of the purée, spreading it all over.
- Top the flatbread with the sliced tomato, followed by the mozzarella slices.
- Sprinkle over the oregano and return to the oven for 8 minutes, until the cheese has melted.
- Once the cheese has melted, remove from the oven and dollop over the pesto evenly. Garnish with the basil leaves.

Lemon Pepper Mayo Fish Finger Butty

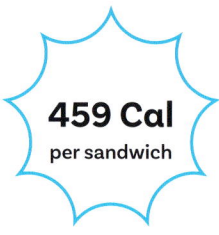

459 Cal per sandwich

| Protein: 36.2g | Fat: 4.9g | Carbs: 58.4g |

SERVES 2

 AF

Let's level up that fish finger sandwich, shall we? Homemade fish fingers are so much nicer than frozen ones in my opinion. These ones are paired with a gorgeous lemon pepper mayo dressing along with some crunchy lettuce, all tucked inside soft white bread. You can use any white fish; it doesn't have to be cod.

Ingredients

2 cod fillets (140g each)
½ tsp garlic granules
½ tsp onion granules
½ tsp paprika
1 tsp plain flour
1 medium egg, whisked
35g panko breadcrumbs
Olive oil spray
4 slices of white bloomer bread (I use Jacksons)
1 little gem lettuce, chopped
Salt and pepper

Sauce
70g lighter than light mayonnaise
1 tbsp lemon juice
½ tsp cracked black pepper
¼ tsp garlic granules
Pinch of salt

Method

- Preheat the air fryer to 185°C.
- Start by patting the cod fillets dry with kitchen paper on both sides.
- Next, slice the fillets into finger shapes by slicing the fillets lengthways and then in half. Crack over a pinch of salt and pepper, then sprinkle over the garlic granules, onion granules, paprika and the flour. Rub gently into the fish fingers.
- Next, dip each finger into the egg wash followed by the breadcrumbs.
- Spray your air fryer basket with a few pumps of olive oil spray. Put each of the fish fingers inside, spraying them with a few pumps of oil. Air fry the fingers for 10–12 minutes.
- While the fish cooks, make the sauce by mixing together all the sauce ingredients.
- Assemble the sandwich by spreading half of the sauce on one side of the bread, top with the cooked fish fingers, followed by the lettuce, and then spread the remaining sauce on the other piece of bread before topping the sandwich.

Oven Preheat the oven to 230°C/210°C fan and bake on a lined baking tray for 15–18 minutes until the fish is flaky, turning partway through.

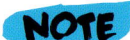

You can make the fingers two long ones if you prefer!

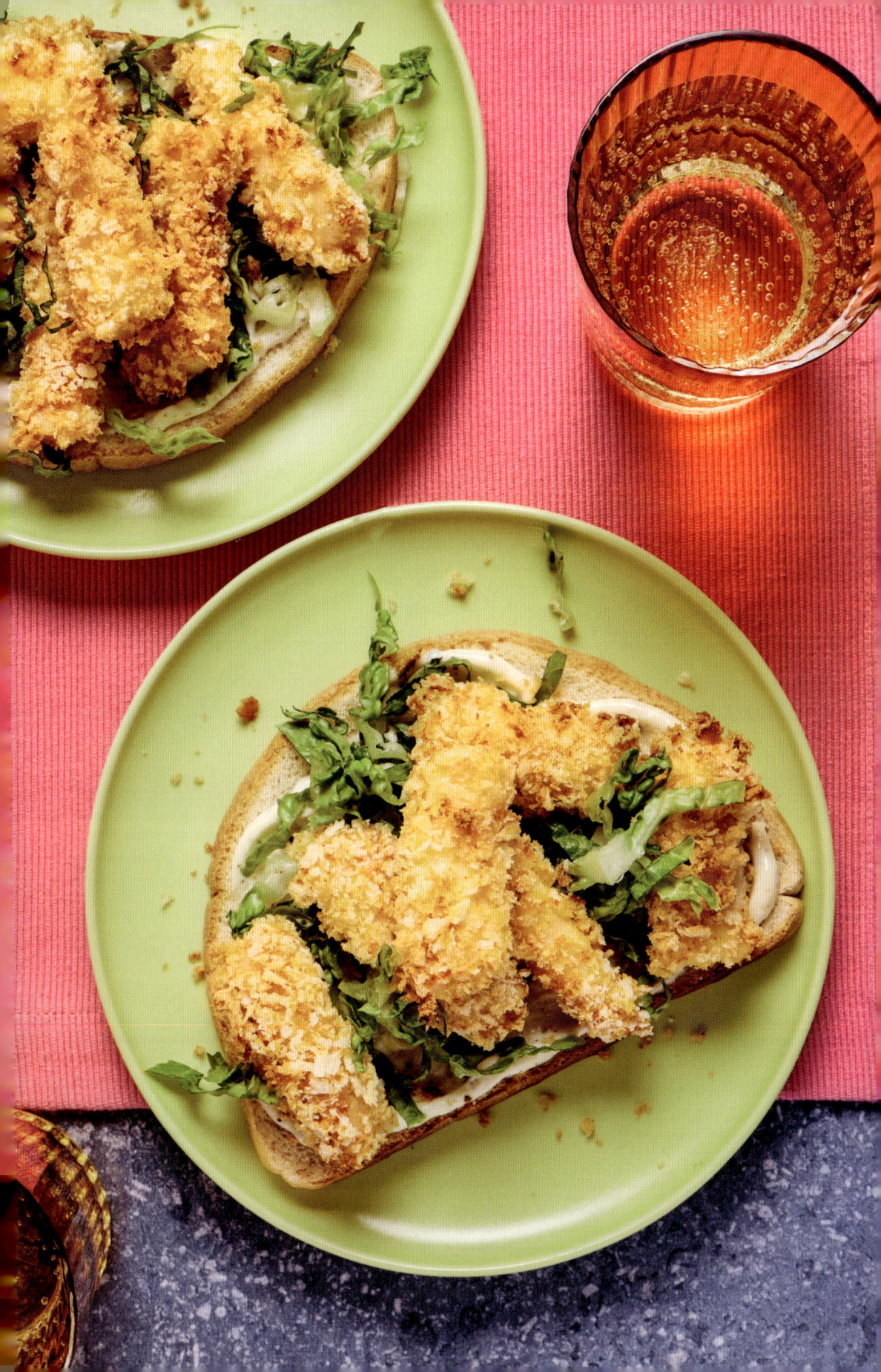

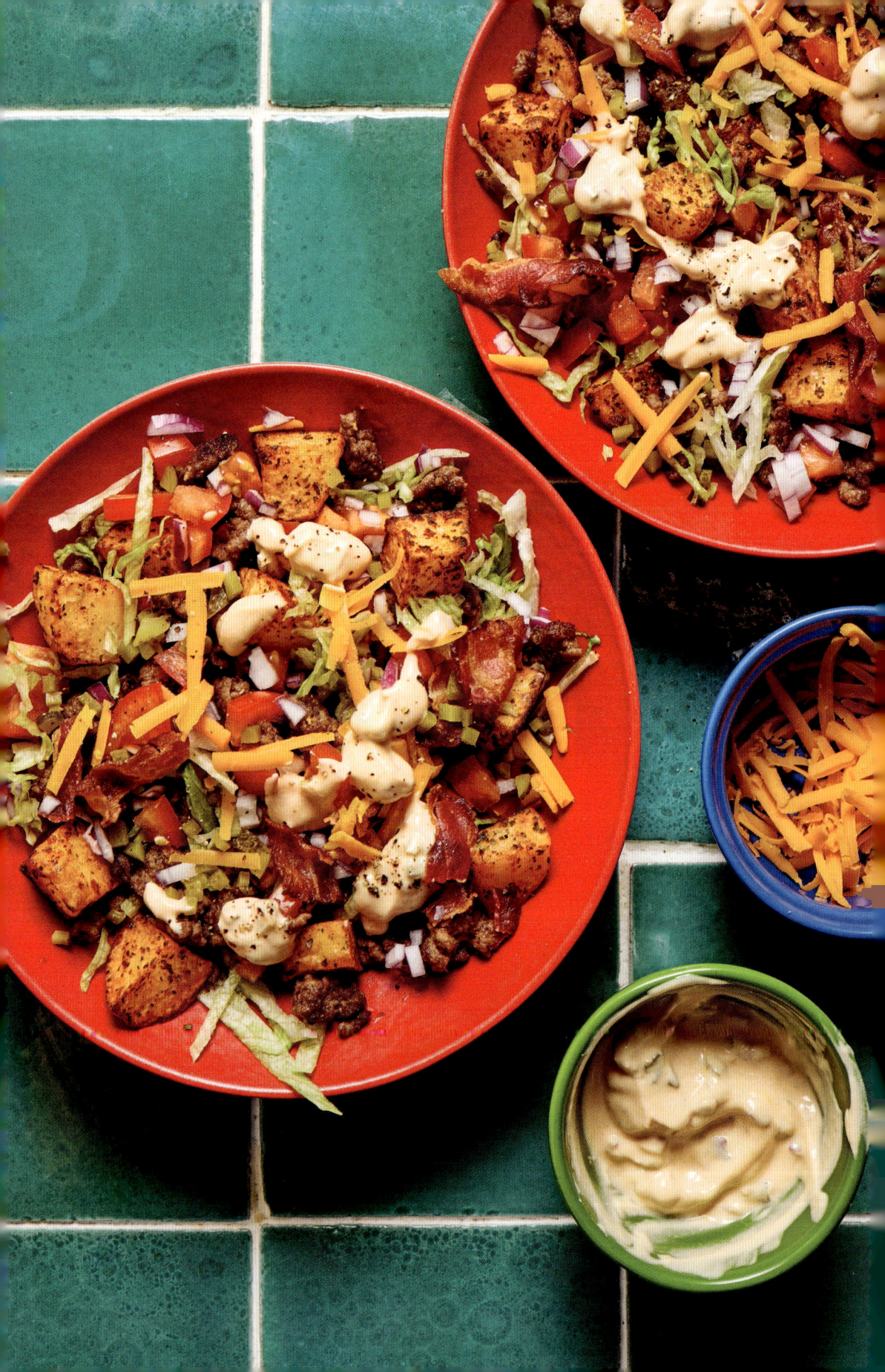

Bacon Cheeseburger Bowls

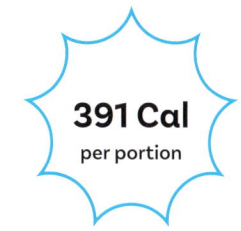

391 Cal per portion

Protein: 38.35g **Fat: 11.4g** **Carbs: 28.95g**

MAKES 2

This is one of my all-time favourite recipes that I rinsed and repeated on my own weight-loss journey. It will definitely keep you full!

Ingredients

250g Maris Piper potato, peeled and cut into 2cm cubes

½ tsp paprika

½ tsp dried parsley

Olive oil spray

200g lean beef mince

1 tsp garlic granules

1 tsp onion granules

2 rashers of streaky bacon

5 baby gherkins, finely chopped

1 red onion, diced

1 tbsp Worcestershire sauce

5 lettuce leaves, chopped

2 salad tomatoes, diced

20g Red Leicester, grated

Salt and pepper

Burger sauce

60g fat-free Greek yoghurt

15g reduced-sugar ketchup

¼ tsp yellow American mustard

Method

- Start by patting the potato dry with kitchen paper and placing it directly into your air fryer drawer. Season with the paprika and parsley along with some salt and pepper. Shake well to distribute the seasonings, spray with a few pumps of olive oil spray and cook for 17 minutes at 200°C, shaking every 5 minutes.

- Preheat the grill to medium-high.

- Next, add the lean beef mince to a medium frying pan, Season with the garlic granules, onion granules and some salt and pepper. Fry for 5-7 minutes, until browned.

- Meanwhile, grill the bacon according to the packet instructions and, once cooked, chop into small pieces.

- Next, make the burger sauce by mixing all the ingredients, and stirring through half the gherkin and a quarter of the red onion, then set to one side.

- Once the beef has browned, add the Worcestershire sauce, mix well and turn off the heat.

- When the potatoes are cooked, assemble the bowls. First add the lettuce, followed by the potatoes, beef, diced tomatoes, Red Leicester, bacon, and the remaining red onion and chopped gherkin. Drizzle over the burger sauce to serve.

Oven Place the potatoes on a baking tray and cook at 220°C/200°C fan for 20-25 minutes, tossing throughout. If taking this on the go, I recommend keeping the sauce in a separate pot.

Gochujang Garlic Bread Cheese Toastie

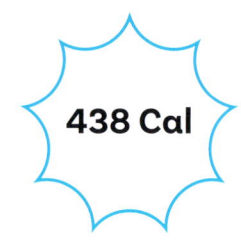

| Protein: 21.8g | Fat: 14.2g | Carbs: 50.9g |

SERVES 1

This is such a banging cheese toastie and a good way to use up gochujang paste! Gochujang adds a delicious peppery, chilli taste that breaks up the creaminess of the soft cheese, Parmesan and mozzarella. Start with the listed amount and add more according to your palate. The toastie is finished with garlic butter for an extra layer of flavour. If you like it, kimchi is another tasty addition.

Ingredients

2 slices of sourdough bread (50g each; I use Jason's)

10g gochujang paste (I use Daesang)

30g lightest cream cheese

5g Parmesan, grated

1 mozzarella slice (the thin slices from a packet), halved

10g light butter

1 tsp chopped garlic

½ tsp dried parsley

Method

- Start by toasting the bread until lightly toasted.
- Meanwhile, heat a dry frying pan over a medium heat.
- In a bowl, mix together the gochujang paste, cream cheese and Parmesan.
- Once the bread is toasted, spread the cream cheese mix over one of the slices. Put the mozzarella on top, along with the other piece of bread and place in the pan. Leave for 2 minutes before flipping.
- While the cheese melts, put the butter, garlic and parsley into a microwavable bowl. Blast in the microwave on high for 10-15 seconds, until melted.
- Cook the toastie for 1 minute, then flip it back over to its original side. Brush half of the garlic butter on this side of the toastie, flip for another 30 seconds and repeat on the other side.
- Remove from the pan and serve.

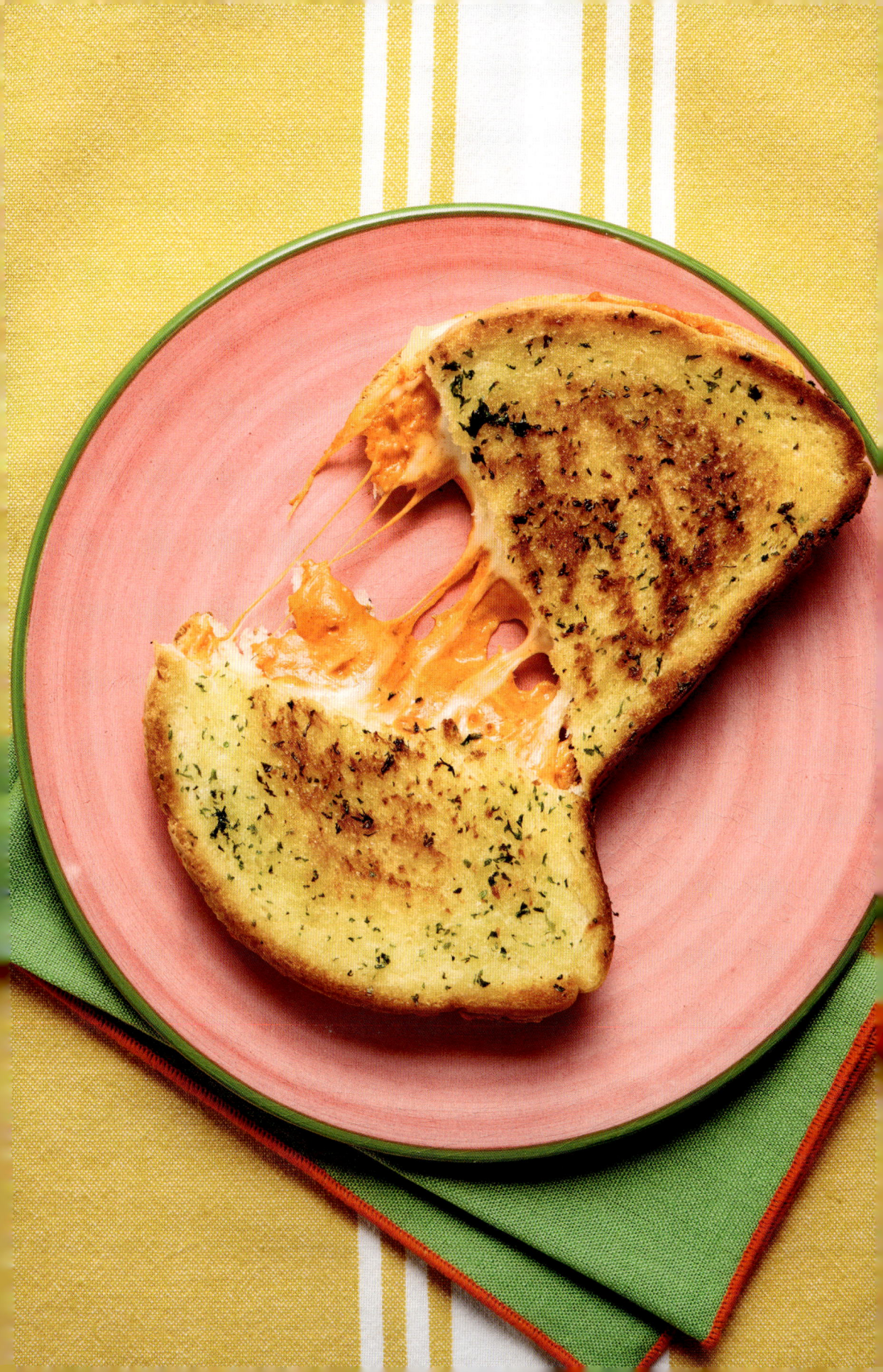

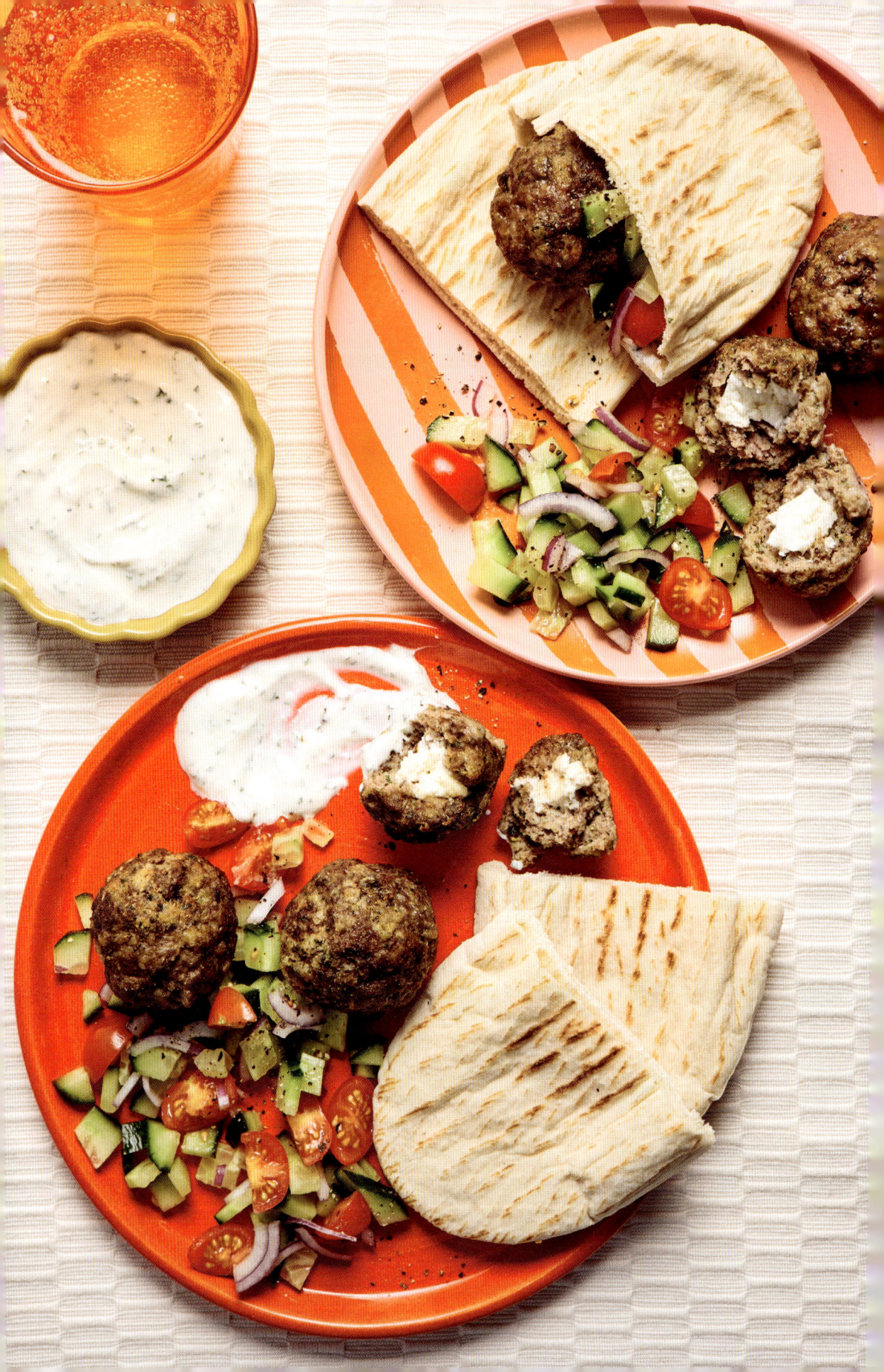

Feta-Stuffed Meatballs

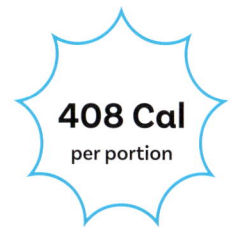
408 Cal per portion

Protein: 44.2g   **Fat: 11g**   **Carbs: 29.6g**

SERVES 2

Who doesn't love a big juicy meatball? Transport yourself to a summer's holiday with these gorgeous feta-stuffed meatballs seasoned with Greek-inspired flavours. Serve them on a bed of garlic herb sauce with toasted pitta bread and chopped salad. Lamb mince also can be used in place of beef and you can always add extra feta to your side salad if you wish.

Ingredients

225g lean beef mince
1 tsp garlic granules
1 tsp onion granules
½ tsp dried oregano
½ tsp dried parsley
¼ tsp dried dill
¼ tsp dried mint
¼ tsp ground cumin
½ medium egg, whisked
20g panko breadcrumbs
30g feta, cut into 6 cubes
Olive oil spray
Salt and pepper

Garlic Herb Sauce

100g fat-free Greek yoghurt
1 tsp chopped garlic
1 tsp lemon juice
½ tsp dried parsley

To serve

2 soft white pitta breads
½ small red onion, diced
4 cherry tomatoes, quartered
½ cucumber, cubed

Method

- Start by heating a large frying pan over a medium heat.
- Next, add all of the ingredients for the meatballs, except the feta, into a bowl and season with salt and pepper. Mix well to combine.
- Use damp hands to split the mixture into 6 equal balls, being careful not to play around with the mixture too much.
- Then, make a small dent in each ball and add a feta cube. Fold the meat back over the feta into a ball shape.
- Spray the frying pan with a few pumps of olive oil spray, then add the stuffed balls and fry over a medium-high heat for 10 minutes, turning the meatballs to brown all of the surface. Then, turn down the heat and cook for a few more minutes, until the balls are cooked through with no pink showing.
- While the meatballs cook, mix the ingredients for the garlic herb sauce with a little salt and set to one side.
- When the meatballs are almost cooked, toast the pitta breads.
- Spread the sauce equally over two plates before topping with the meatballs. Serve the onion, tomatoes and cucumber tossed together on the side along with the toasted pitta breads.

Four

BATCH COOK

Halloumi Curry

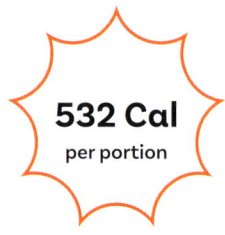

532 Cal per portion

Protein: 29.5g **Fat: 23.3g** **Carbs: 58.6g**

SERVES 2

This is one of my all-time favourite veggie curries. Bites of halloumi are pan-fried until golden and tossed into an easy homemade curry sauce along with chopped spinach. You can use paneer if you prefer, or chicken for a non-veggie version.

Ingredients

2 × 125g packets of boil-in-the-bag long-grain rice

Olive oil spray

1 white onion, diced

1 tsp chopped garlic

1 tsp ginger purée

1½ tsp ground cumin

1 tsp ground turmeric

1 tsp ground coriander

1 tsp mild chilli powder

1½ tsp garam masala

1 × 400g tin of chopped tomatoes

1 vegetable stock cube

200ml hot water

350g reduced-fat halloumi, cubed

90ml reduced-fat single cream alternative (I use Elmlea)

1 tsp granulated sweetener

2 handfuls of spinach, chopped

A few sprigs of fresh coriander, chopped

Salt and pepper

Method

- Start by cooking the rice in a large pan of water according to the packet instructions.

- Next, spray a large frying pan with a few pumps of olive oil spray. Over a high heat, add the onion, garlic and ginger. Sauté for a couple of minutes until the onion has softened.

- Next, add the cumin, turmeric, coriander, chilli powder and garam masala, along with salt and pepper to taste. Mix well before adding the chopped tomatoes, stock cube and hot water. Leave over a medium heat to thicken.

- Once the sauce has reduced slightly, put the halloumi into a separate clean pan and cook for 4–5 minutes, until golden.

- Add the cream and sweetener to the curry sauce, mixing well before adding the chopped spinach. Leave on the heat for a few minutes until the spinach has wilted slightly, then stir in the cooked halloumi.

- Remove from the heat and serve over the freshly cooked rice, scattered with the coriander.

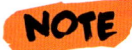

If you can't get the reduced-fat cream alternative, you can use half the amount of normal cream and half semi-skimmed milk. Make sure to use both at room temperature and always increase heat slowly to avoid the sauce separating.

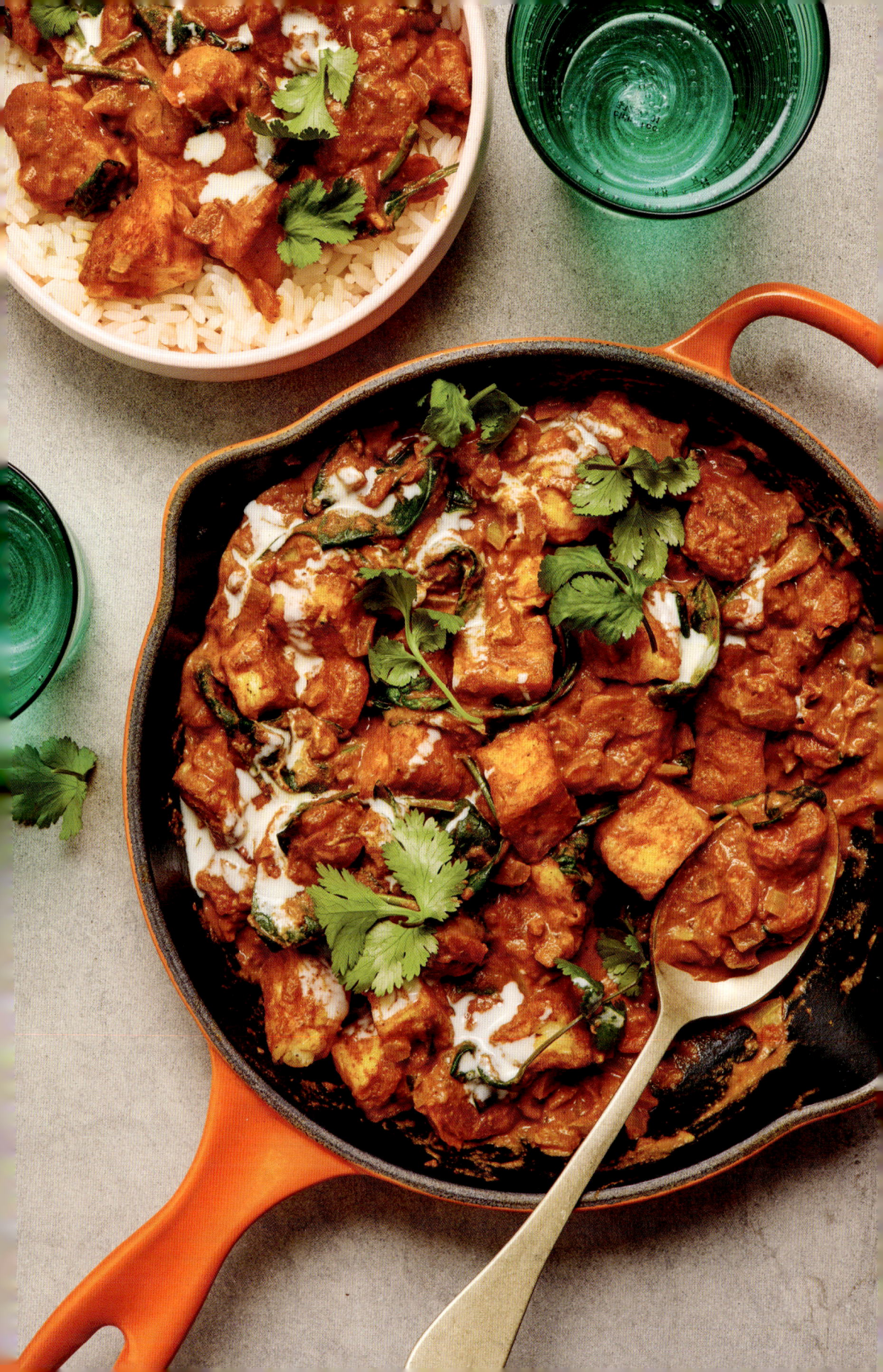

Swedish Meatballs and Mash

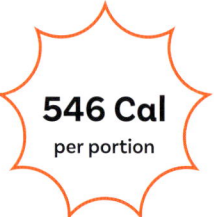

546 Cal per portion

Protein: 44.2g Fat: 14.7g Carbs: 49.9g

SERVES 4

AF

No more waiting around for that trip to buy furniture, you can make your own version at home!

Ingredients

800g Maris Piper potatoes, peeled and cut into 2.5cm cubes
500g lean beef mince
1 tsp onion granules
1 tsp garlic granules
1 medium egg
20g panko breadcrumbs
Olive oil spray
120ml semi-skimmed milk
15g light butter
Salt and pepper
A few sprigs of fresh parsley, chopped, to garnish

Sauce

20g light butter
15g plain flour
400ml hot beef stock
½ tsp garlic granules
1 tsp dark soy sauce
1 tbsp Worcestershire sauce
½ tsp Dijon mustard
100g light cream cheese

Method

- Preheat the oven to 230°C/210°C fan.
- Put the potatoes into a large pan of salted boiling water and cook for 14–15 minutes or until tender when you prod them with a fork.
- Put the beef into a bowl and season with the onion granules, garlic granules and some salt and pepper. Crack in the egg and add the breadcrumbs. Combine the mixture.
- Spray a large baking tray with a few pumps of olive oil. Roll 16 meatballs out of the beef mixture, transferring each to the baking tray. Place in the oven for 10 minutes, turning partway through.
- While they cook, make the sauce by putting the butter into a saucepan over a medium heat. Once melted, add the flour and stir continuously with a whisk for 2 minutes. Once a roux (a thick paste) has formed, gradually pour in the beef stock in 100ml increments, whisking continuously to achieve a smooth sauce.
- Once all of the beef stock is in the pan, turn up the heat slightly. Add the garlic granules, soy sauce, Worcestershire sauce and mustard.
- When the stock has reduced slightly, add the cream cheese and leave to thicken. (Please note, once removed from the heat, the sauce will thicken further.)
- Once the potatoes are done, drain, return them to the pan and add the milk and butter. Season with salt and pepper to taste. Using a potato masher, mash the potatoes until smooth. If you have an electric hand whisk, you can use this to achieve a super-smooth mash.
- Serve the mashed potatoes with the meatballs on top. Pour over the creamy sauce and scatter over the fresh parsley.

Air fryer Air fry the meatballs for 10 minutes at 180°C, turning partway through.

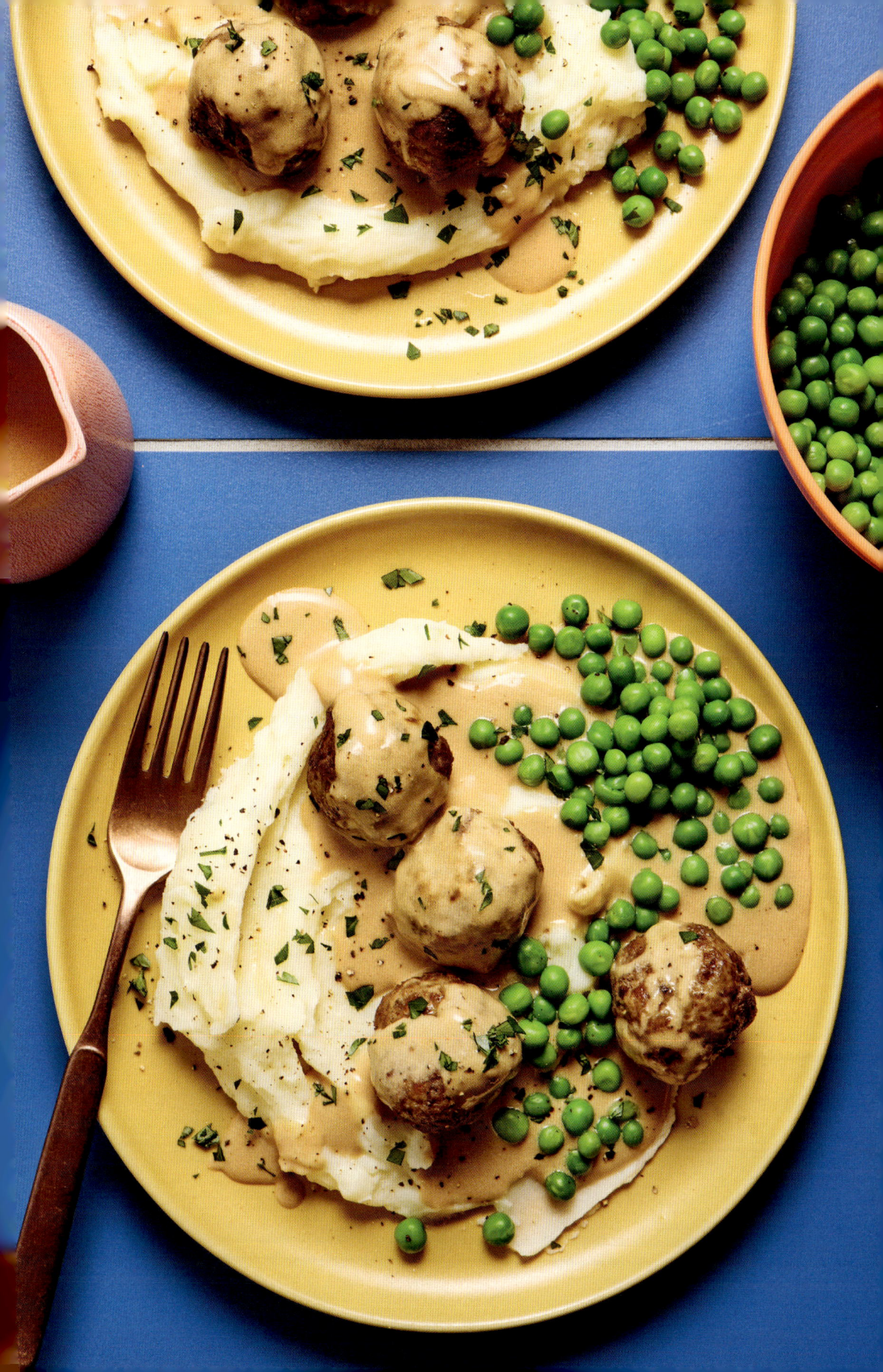

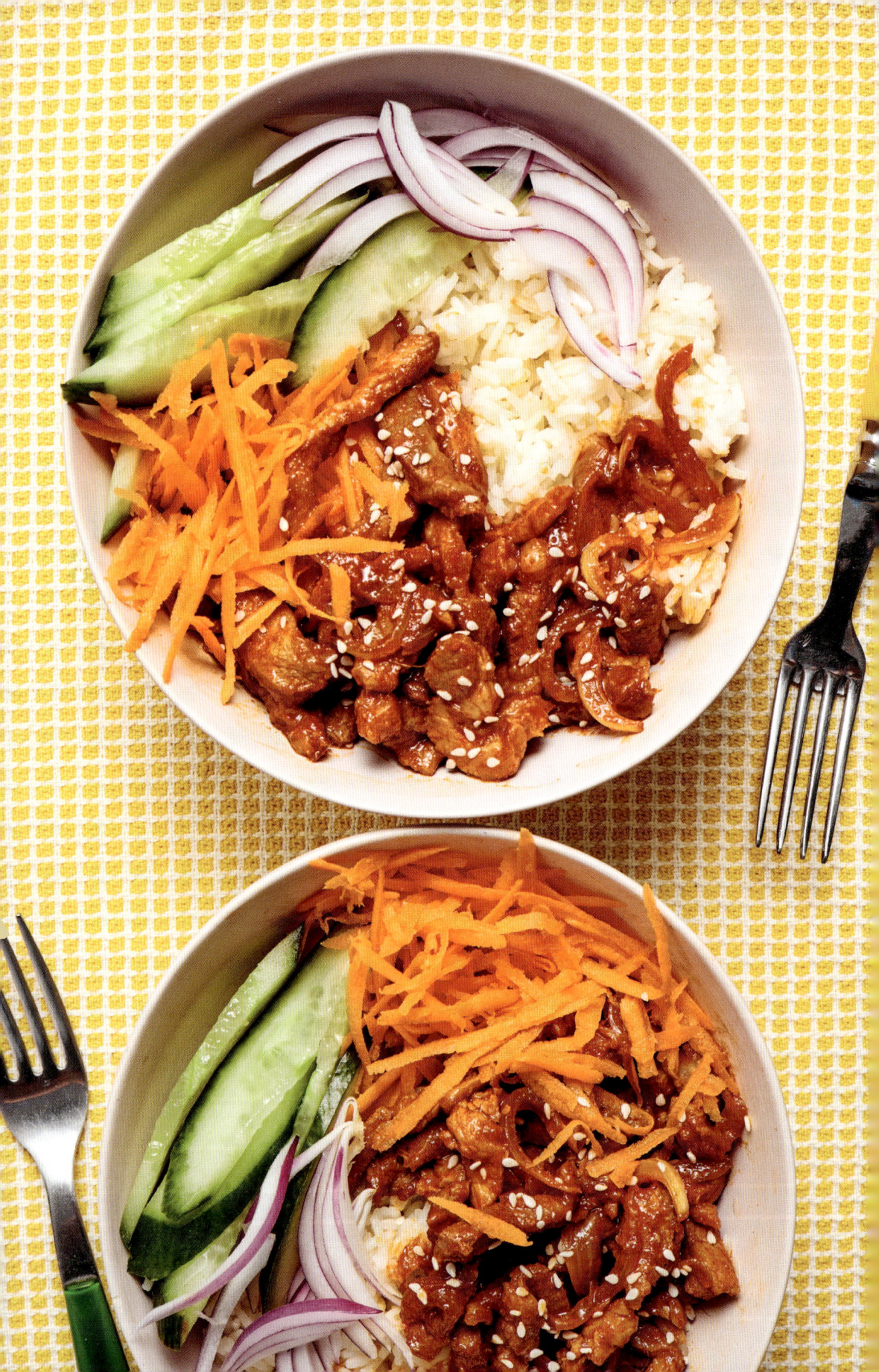

Gochujang BBQ Pork Bowls

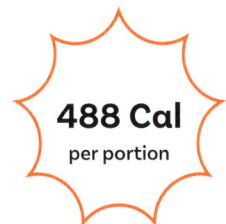

488 Cal per portion

| Protein: 41.7g | Fat: 10.3g | Carbs: 54.1g |

SERVES 4

This recipe is so easy to make yet it tastes incredible. The pork is bold in flavour, while the veggies in the bowl help to keep things nice and fresh. If you do have the time to marinate your pork, it helps to deepen the flavours, but don't worry if you don't – it is still banging. You can pack these bowls with anything you like: avocado is yummy for added fats, or you can throw in some kimchi for a kick of gut-health support.

Ingredients

400g lean pork stir-fry strips

1 white onion, sliced

1 tsp smoked paprika

1 tsp garlic granules

2 tsp sesame oil

25g gochujang paste (I use Daesang)

60ml light soy sauce

1 tbsp oyster sauce (can substitute for honey)

2 tsp chopped garlic

1 tsp chopped ginger

2 tbsp rice vinegar

2 × 250g packets of microwave jasmine rice

1 cucumber, sliced

1 medium carrot, grated

1 red onion, sliced

1 tsp sesame seeds, to garnish

Method

- Start by putting the pork into a large bowl along with the onion. Next, add the smoked paprika, garlic granules, a teaspoon of the sesame oil, the gochujang paste, light soy sauce, oyster sauce, garlic, ginger and rice vinegar. Mix well to combine.
- Heat a large frying pan and add the remaining teaspoon of sesame oil.
- Once the oil is hot, add the pork and all of its marinade and fry for 8 minutes over a high heat, until cooked through.
- While the pork cooks, microwave the packets of rice.
- Once cooked, divide the rice equally between your bowls. Add the cucumber, carrot and red onion. When the pork is cooked, add it to the bowl of rice and garnish with the sesame seeds.

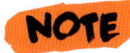

If you are unable to get pork stir-fry strips, you can use thin pork loin steaks and cut them into strips. If you prefer crispier pork, you can pan-fry it first then pour over the sauce.

Aubergine Parmigiana

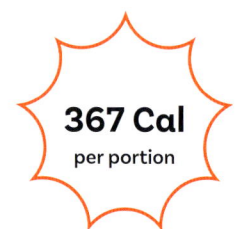

Protein: 16.8g **Fat: 14.8g** **Carbs: 26.4g**

SERVES 2

I usually steer clear of aubergine on a busy weeknight just because it can be a faff to make. However, with the use of a microwave it's ready in just a fraction of the time. Layered with a pesto passata mix, mozzarella, garlic breadcrumbs and Parmesan, it's a seriously delicious veggie dinner.

Ingredients

2 medium aubergines

10g light butter

1 tsp chopped garlic

20g panko breadcrumbs

20g Parmesan, grated

30g reduced-fat red pesto

200g good-quality passata

1 tsp oregano

100g light mozzarella, sliced

Salt and pepper

A few fresh basil leaves, to garnish

Method

- Start by preheating the oven to 240°C/220°C fan.
- Prick the aubergines all over with a fork or a toothpick. Place on a microwavable plate and cook on full power for 7 minutes.
- While the aubergines are cooking, put the butter into a small frying pan. Once melted, add the garlic and breadcrumbs. Cook for 3–4 minutes over a medium heat until the breadcrumbs are golden all over. Remove from the heat and add the Parmesan.
- Once the time is up on the aubergines, turn them carefully (they will be hot) and cook for a further 2 minutes, until tender.
- Meanwhile, put the pesto and passata into a bowl. Season with salt and pepper, add the oregano and give the mixture a good stir.
- Once the aubergines are cooked, carefully remove the plate from the microwave (I like to use an oven glove).
- Slice off the ends of the aubergines and cut them lengthways down the middle.
- Transfer to a large baking dish. Top with the passata mixture, followed by the sliced mozzarella and breadcrumb mix.
- Bake in the oven for 5 minutes until the cheese has melted, then remove and serve.

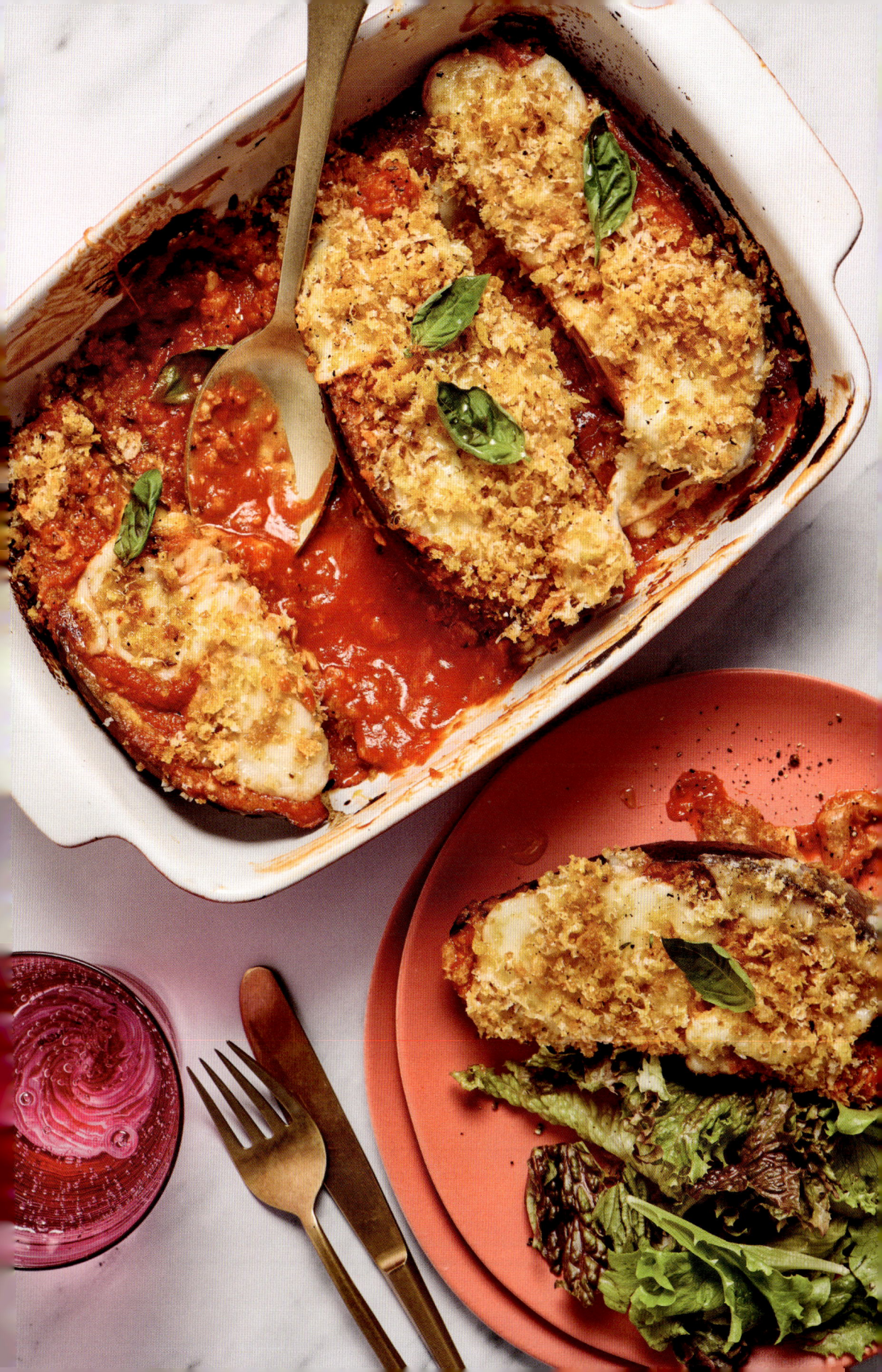

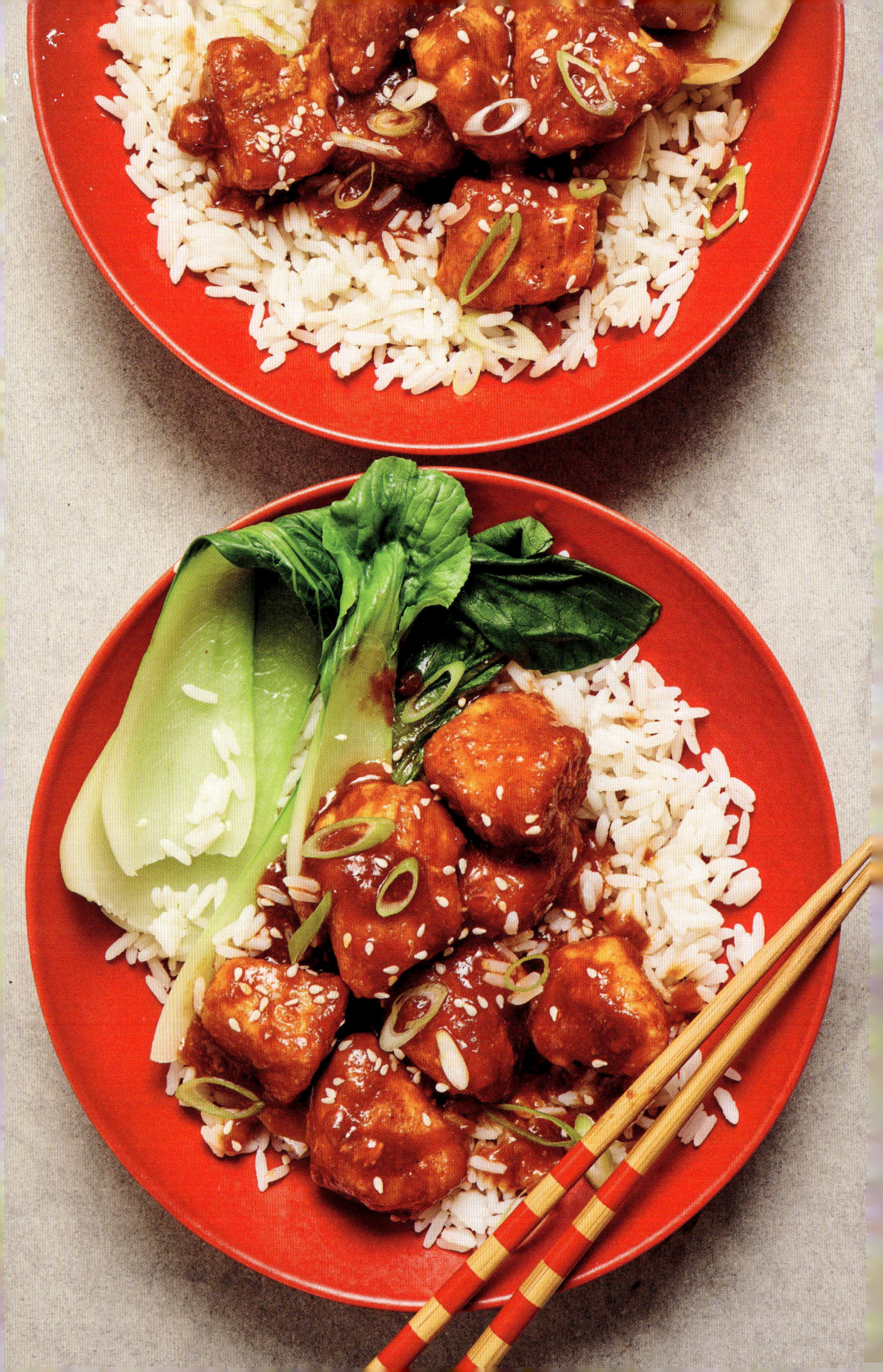

Sweet Chilli Glazed Chicken Bites

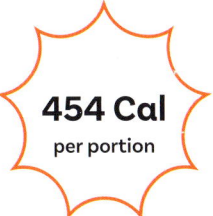

454 Cal per portion

| Protein: 39.9g | Fat: 3.9g | Carbs: 63.6g |

SERVES 4

Tender pieces of chicken are tossed in the most delicious sticky sweet chilli glaze. I like to pair this with some pan-fried pak choi or broccoli, to add some veggies, and I serve it over noodles when I fancy a change.

Ingredients

2 × 125g packets of boil-in-the-bag rice

500g skinless chicken breast, cut into 2.5cm cubes

1 tsp paprika

1 tsp garlic granules

10g cornflour

Olive oil spray

2 spring onions, sliced

1 tsp sesame seeds

Sauce

45g reduced-sugar ketchup

50ml light soy sauce

90g reduced-sugar sweet chilli sauce

1 tbsp rice wine vinegar

1 tsp chopped garlic

1 tsp chopped ginger

Method

- Start by cooking the rice according to the packet instructions.
- Next, season the chicken with the paprika, garlic granules and cornflour. Mix well to combine.
- Spray a large frying pan with a few pumps of olive oil spray.
- Place the pan over a medium-high heat and add the chicken, ensuring it is not overlapping. Fry for 8–9 minutes, until cooked through.
- While the chicken cooks, mix together the sauce ingredients and set to one side.
- When the chicken has cooked through, turn the heat down to low. Pour in the sauce and leave for 2 minutes. If you want a thinner sauce, you can splash 2 tablespoons of water into the pan directly.
- Drain the rice and divide equally between bowls. Top with the cooked chicken, followed by the spring onions and sesame seeds.

Air Fryer Air fry the chicken for 10 minutes at 190°C.

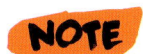

This will keep in the fridge for up to 4 days. When reheating, you can add a dash of water or stock to the bites to allow the sauce to loosen.

Tandoori Chicken Rice Bowls

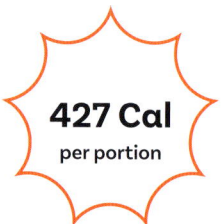

427 Cal per portion

Protein: 36.6g **Fat: 5.2g** **Carbs: 52.5g**

SERVES 4

 AF

Light, fresh and absolutely banging – you will love these flavoursome tandoori bowls!

Ingredients

400g skinless chicken breast, cut into 2.5cm cubes

2 tbsp tandoori seasoning

1 tbsp lemon juice

1 tbsp fat-free natural yoghurt

1–2 tsp red food colouring (optional)

Olive oil spray

200g lettuce, shredded

4 salad tomatoes, diced

1 small red onion, diced

1 small cucumber, diced

2 × 250g packets of microwave basmati rice

2 mini garlic and coriander naan breads

Garlic and coriander sauce

80g fat-free natural yoghurt

1 tsp chopped garlic

1 tsp lemon juice

2 sprigs of fresh coriander, chopped

Pinch of salt

Method

- Preheat the oven to 220°C/200°C fan.
- Put the chicken into a bowl and season with the tandoori seasoning. Add the lemon juice, natural yoghurt and food colouring, if using, and give everything a good stir.
- Thread the chicken onto metal skewers. If you have wooden skewers, ensure that you soak them for 30 minutes prior to cooking to prevent them from burning.
- Place on a non-stick baking tray, spray the tray with a few pumps of olive oil spray and cook for 14 minutes, basting with the juices partway through.
- While the chicken cooks, mix all the ingredients for the garlic and coriander sauce and set to one side.
- Next, build the bowls with the lettuce, tomatoes, red onion and cucumber.
- When there are a few minutes left of the chicken cooking time, microwave the rice according to the packet instructions and divide it between your bowls.
- Next, chop the naan breads into triangle shapes. Drizzle with water and place on a non-stick baking tray. Cook for 2–3 minutes, until slightly crispy.
- Meanwhile, to get extra char on the skewers, transfer to a hot grill for a further minute or two.
- Add the skewers to the bowls, drizzle over the garlic and coriander yoghurt sauce and top with the crispy naan triangles.

Air fryer Cook the chicken for the same amount of time at 200°C. Cook the naan chips at 185°C for 2 minutes, turning partway.

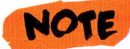

If you're meal prepping, store the sauce separately and add the salad fresh. If taking the bowl on the go, I like to put the salad into a ziplock bag.

Cheesy Chipotle Beef Pasta

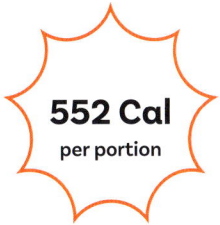

552 Cal per portion

Protein: 43.8g **Fat: 13.8g** **Carbs: 55.2g**

SERVES 4

This is one of my favourite pastas for when you need a dinner that you know is going to really hit the spot, plus it tastes really good reheated so leftovers are perfect. A sweet and smoky beef mince is paired with Red Leicester cheese and mozzarella, which are the perfect combination for the flavours within the pasta. You can sub the mozzarella for low-fat cheddar if you wish. This would be veggie friendly if you use quorn mince instead of the beef, and a vegetable stock cube.

Ingredients

250g dried pasta
Olive oil spray
400g lean beef mince
1 red onion, diced
1 red pepper, diced
1½ tsp oregano
1 tsp smoked paprika
2 tsp chopped garlic
30g runny honey
2 tsp chipotle paste
1 tbsp tomato purée
4 tbsp tomato salsa
1 beef stock cube, crumbled
40g Red Leicester, grated
80g mozzarella, grated
A few sprigs of fresh parsley, chopped
A few chilli flakes (optional)

Method

- Start by cooking the pasta in a large pan of salted water according to the packet instructions, removing 200ml of the cooking water towards the end of the cooking time and setting aside for the sauce.
- Preheat the grill to high.
- Spray a large frying pan with a few pumps of olive oil spray, place over a high heat, add the beef mince and fry for 4–5 minutes, until browned.
- Once browned, add the onion and red pepper and fry for a couple more minutes, until softened.
- When the veggies are soft, add the oregano, smoked paprika and chopped garlic and fry for an additional 30 seconds. Squeeze in the honey, before adding the chipotle paste, tomato purée, salsa, stock cube and the reserved pasta water.
- Combine the cooked pasta with the mince, then top with both types of cheese before placing underneath the hot grill.
- Once the cheese has melted, remove from the grill and garnish with the fresh parsley and chilli flakes, if using.

Sticky Sesame Chicken on Noodles

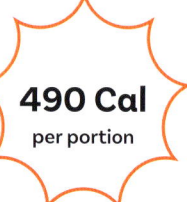

490 Cal per portion

Protein: 36.8g **Fat: 8.8g** **Carbs: 62.47g**

SERVES 4

 DF

Dinner never tasted so damn good and guilt free: golden pieces of chicken coated in a sweet, sticky and tangy sauce paired with noodles for a delicious, healthy dinner. Serve with steamed Tenderstem broccoli or pak choi or throw some prawn crackers on the side.

Ingredients

1 tbsp sesame oil

400g skinless chicken breast, cut into 2.5cm cubes

1 tsp paprika

1 tsp garlic granules

25g cornflour

4 medium egg noodle nests

2½ tbsp dark soy sauce

2 spring onions, sliced

50ml hot water

Salt and pepper

2 tsp sesame seeds, to garnish

Sauce

1 tbsp sesame oil

50g reduced-sugar ketchup

45g reduced-sugar sweet chilli sauce

40g runny honey

2 tbsp rice vinegar

20ml light soy sauce

1 tsp chopped garlic

1 tsp brown sugar

Method

- Start by adding the sesame oil to a large frying pan set over a high heat.
- Put the chicken into a bowl, then season with the paprika, garlic granules and some salt and pepper to taste. Add the cornflour and mix well to ensure the chicken pieces are coated.
- Add the chicken pieces to the pan and cook over a high heat for 8-10 minutes, until golden and cooked through. Keep moving the chicken pieces around to prevent them burning.
- While the chicken cooks, mix the sauce ingredients in a bowl and set to one side.
- Cook the noodle nests as per the packet instructions, then drain and rinse with cold water to prevent them from sticking together. Return them to the pan and pour in 2 tablespoons of the sauce along with the dark soy sauce and half the spring onions, mixing to ensure they are coated well.
- Pour the remaining sauce into the pan with the chicken, add the water and stir to coat the chicken pieces. Cook for 2 minutes over a medium heat, until slightly reduced.
- Serve the cooked noodles in a bowl with the chicken on top. Garnish with the remaining spring onion and the sesame seeds.

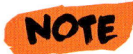

Check the nutritional information on the noodle packet to find the ones that are lowest in calories.

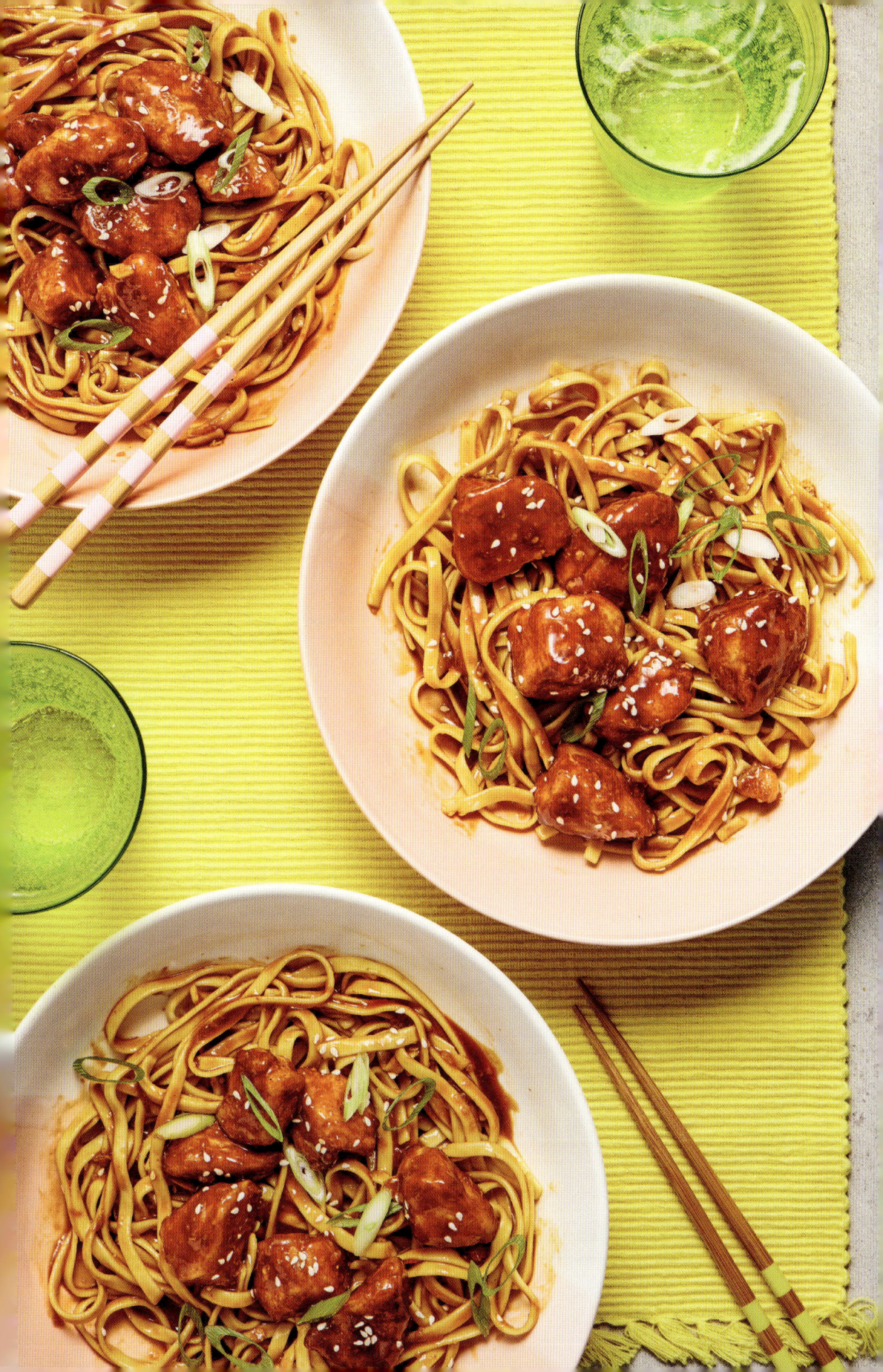

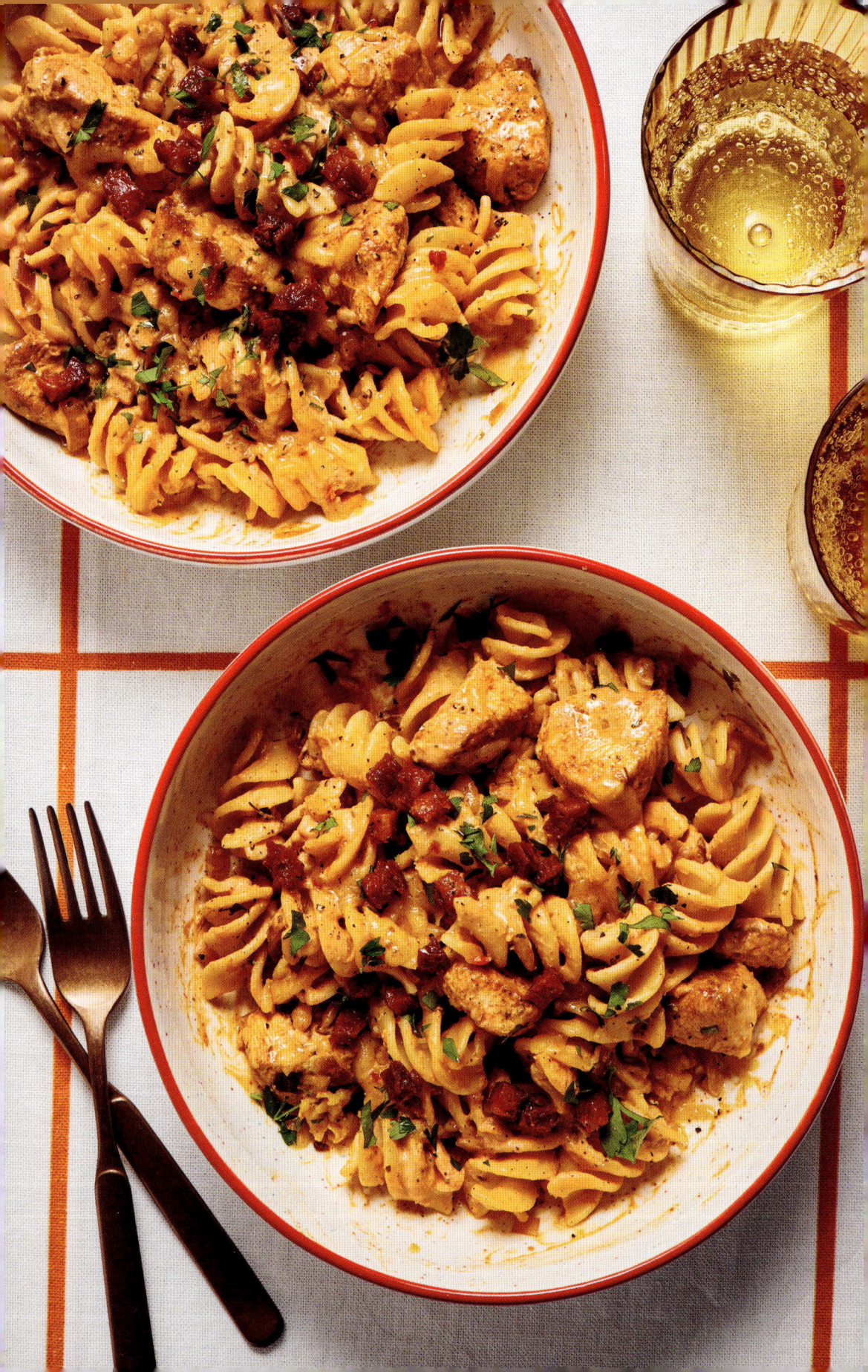

Cheesy Chicken and Chorizo Pasta

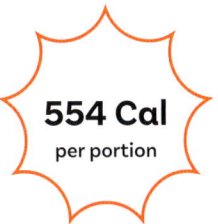

554 Cal per portion

Protein: 47.3g **Fat: 16.9g** **Carbs: 47.6g**

SERVES 4

This pasta dish is going to be a huge hit at dinner time. Inspired by Mexican flavours, it's so delicious.

Ingredients

Olive oil spray

60g chorizo, diced

400g skinless chicken breast, cut into 2.5cm cubes

1 tbsp + ½ tsp smoked paprika

½ tbsp + ½ tsp dried oregano

240g dried pasta

1 large red onion, diced

2 tsp chopped garlic

2 tbsp tomato purée

100g reduced-fat garlic and herb cream cheese

80g Mexican cheese, grated (you can substitute this for chipotle cheddar or Red Leicester)

Salt and pepper

A few sprigs of fresh parsley, chopped, to garnish

Method

- Spray a large frying pan with a few pumps of olive oil spray. Over a high heat, fry off the chorizo for 3 minutes.
- Meanwhile, season the chicken with the tablespoon of smoked paprika and the half tablespoon of oregano, along with some salt and pepper. Rub in thoroughly.
- Cook the pasta in a large pan of salted water according to the packet instructions, removing 170ml of the cooking water towards the end of the cooking time and setting aside for the sauce.
- Remove the chorizo from the pan, leaving behind its oil, and transfer it to a bowl. Add the cubed chicken to the pan and fry for 6 minutes, until almost cooked, before adding the onion for a further 2 minutes.
- Next, add the chopped garlic for 30 seconds and then the tomato purée and cream cheese.
- Mix well before adding the reserved pasta water and remaining half teaspoons of smoked paprika and oregano. Leave over a medium-high heat until the sauce has thickened.
- Once the pasta is cooked, drain and combine with the chicken and sauce. Top with the grated cheese followed by the chorizo. Place under the grill for two minutes until the cheese has melted. Alternatively, you can leave it on the hob over a medium heat, covered with a lid, to melt the cheese.
- Finish by scattering the parsley all over.

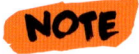

This recipe will keep in the fridge for up to 3 days. To reheat, simply place in a microwavable container and heat for 2-3 minutes, until hot all the way through. To loosen the sauce, I recommend adding a tablespoon or two of water.

Creamy Parmesan Cajun Chicken and Rice

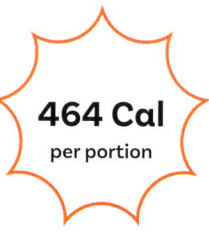

464 Cal per portion

Protein: 37.65g **Fat: 11.17g** **Carbs: 48g**

SERVES 4

This recipe was loved by lots of you when I first shared it on social media. With a few tweaks I've managed to get the cooking time down to under 20 minutes!

Ingredients

2 × 125g packets of boil-in-the-bag long-grain rice (I use Tesco's)

Olive oil spray

400g skinless chicken breast, cut into 2cm cubes

4½ tsp Cajun seasoning

10g light butter

2 heaped tsp chopped garlic

2 shallots, finely diced

1½ tsp Italian herb seasoning

150ml reduced-fat single cream alternative (I use Elmlea)

300ml hot chicken stock (made with 2 cubes)

30g Parmesan, grated

1 tsp garlic granules

Salt and pepper

A few sprigs of fresh parsley, chopped, to garnish

Method

- Start by adding the bags of rice to a large pan of boiling water and cook according to the packet instructions.
- Spray a large frying pan with a few pumps of olive oil spray and place over a medium-high heat.
- While the pan heats, season the chicken with 1½ teaspoons of the Cajun seasoning along with some salt and pepper. Transfer to the pan and cook over a high heat for around 8 minutes, until cooked through.
- Once the chicken has cooked, remove it, and all its juices, from the pan. Next, add the butter, garlic and shallot to the pan and fry for a couple of minutes or until the shallot has softened.
- Add another 2 teaspoons of the Cajun seasoning along with a teaspoon of the Italian herb seasoning. Mix well, before adding the cream and 200ml of the chicken stock. Leave over a medium-high heat, stirring continuously, until thickened.
- When there is a minute left on the rice, stir the grated Parmesan through the sauce and turn the heat down low.
- Drain all the water from the rice pan, then empty the bags of rice into the pan. Season with the remaining teaspoon of Cajun seasoning, the remaining half teaspoon of Italian herb seasoning and the garlic granules. Mix well before pouring in the remaining 100ml of stock and a ladle of the sauce. Return the pan to a medium heat and stir for 30 seconds, until the sauce has evaporated, then take it off the hob.
- Return the chicken and its juices to the frying pan and stir into the sauce. Once combined, take off the hob.
- Serve the seasoned rice with the chicken and sauce over the top. Garnish with the fresh parsley to finish.

Singapore-Style Noodles

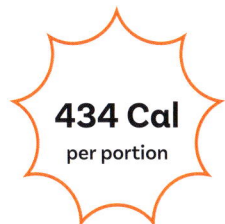
434 Cal per portion

Protein: 37.1g **Fat: 7.6g** **Carbs: 48.7g**

SERVES 4

This is one of my favourite go-to weight-loss recipes; it feels a little cheeky but it definitely isn't. Try prawn, pork or tofu as alternatives to the chicken.

Ingredients

Neutral cooking spray
400g skinless chicken breast, cut into 2.5cm cubes
½ tbsp curry powder
2 medium eggs, whisked
1 onion, thinly sliced
1 red pepper, thinly sliced
150g beansprouts
2 tsp chopped garlic
2 tsp ginger purée
2 × 150g packets of ready-to-wok rice noodles
50–100ml hot water, to loosen
50g curry sauce concentrate mixed with 100ml hot water (I use Goldfish)
1 spring onion, chopped

Sauce
4 tbsp light soy sauce
3 tsp mild curry powder
1½ tsp ground turmeric
½ tsp brown sugar
2 tbsp rice wine vinegar

Method

- Start by spraying a large wok with cooking spray and placing it over a high heat.
- While the wok heats, season the chicken with the curry powder. Mix, then add the chicken to the wok and cook for 7–8 minutes, until cooked through. Remove from the pan and transfer to a plate.
- Make the sauce by combining the soy sauce, curry powder, turmeric, brown sugar and rice wine vinegar and set to one side.
- Turn down the heat under the wok to medium and add the whisked eggs. Leave for 30 seconds to set slightly before pushing them around in the pan to scramble them. You want to take them out of the pan when they are still slightly wet. Add to the plate with the chicken.
- Spray the wok with more cooking spray, then add the onion, red pepper and beansprouts. Pan-fry for 2 minutes before adding the garlic and ginger and frying for a further 30 seconds. Next, add the rice noodles for a further 2 minutes.
- Push the noodles to one side and pour in the water – start with 50ml and increase as needed to loosen the noodles, then mix in the chicken and egg and remove the wok from the heat.
- Put the curry concentrate and water into a saucepan over a high heat. Stir continuously for 1 minute, until thickened, then remove from the heat.
- Serve the noodles with the curry sauce drizzled over, along with the chopped spring onion.

Smoky Sausage 'Casserole' with Cheesy Garlic Bread

492 Cal per portion

Protein: 25.8g   Fat: 19.5g   Carbs: 46.7g

SERVES 4

Okay, I use the word 'casserole' loosely here but this recipe certainly gives those comforting vibes without taking lots of time.

Ingredients

Olive oil spray
8 reduced-fat pork sausages
4 small part-baked rolls
1 red onion, finely sliced
1 red pepper, diced
2 celery sticks, diced
4 tsp chopped garlic
1 tsp ground cumin
1 tsp smoked paprika
1 tsp chipotle paste
1 tbsp Worcestershire sauce
1 beef stock cube
1½ × 400g tins of chopped tomatoes (600g in total)
200ml water
20g light butter
1 tsp dried parsley
60g reduced-fat cheddar, grated
Salt and pepper
A few sprigs of fresh coriander, chopped, to garnish

Method

- Preheat the oven according to the packet instructions for the bread rolls.
- Start by spraying a large frying pan with a few pumps of olive oil spray. Over a high heat, fry the sausages for 12 minutes or until cooked through.
- Place the bread rolls in the oven and bake according to the packet instructions.
- Meanwhile, heat a second pan with a few sprays of olive oil spray. Over a medium heat, sauté the onion, red pepper and celery for around 5 minutes until they have softened.
- When the veggies are soft, add 2 teaspoons of the chopped garlic for 30 seconds, before adding the cumin, smoked paprika and some salt and pepper. Give it all a good mix, then add the chipotle paste and Worcestershire sauce, crumble over the beef stock cube and add the chopped tomatoes and water. Leave to simmer over a medium heat.
- In a small bowl, mix together the remaining garlic with the butter and parsley. When they're ready, carefully cut the rolls in half before brushing the garlic butter over each cut side. Top with the grated cheddar and return to the oven for 5 minutes.
- Once the sausages are cooked, add them to the pan of tomatoes and stir to combine. Leave to simmer for a further 2 minutes, then remove from the heat.
- Serve in bowls, with the fresh coriander on top and the cheesy garlic rolls on the side for dipping.

Slow cooker You can make this recipe in a slow cooker. Brown the sausages before adding all of the remaining casserole ingredients. Cook on low for 7 hours or on high for 4.

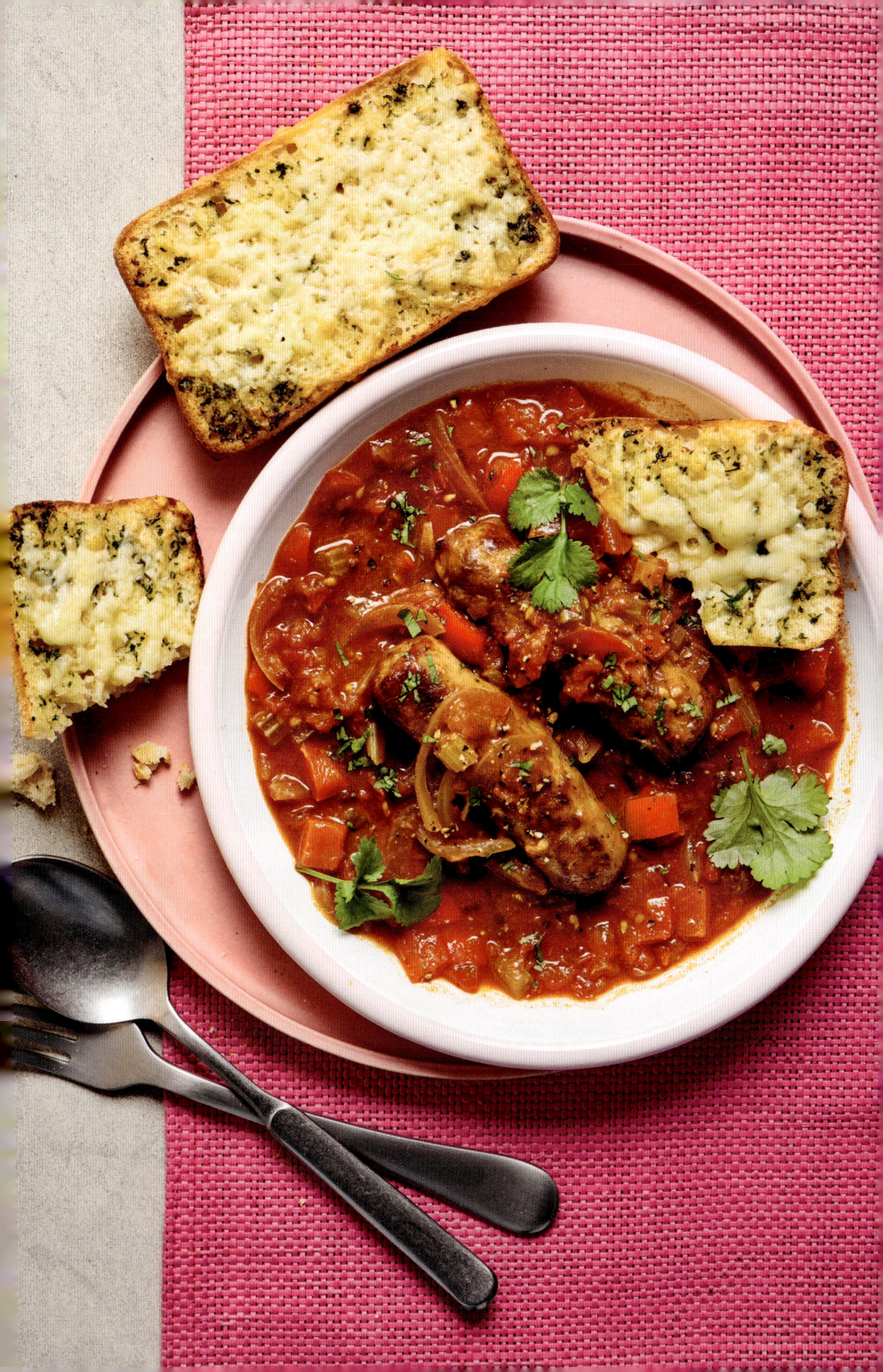

Sweet and Sticky Pork Fried Rice

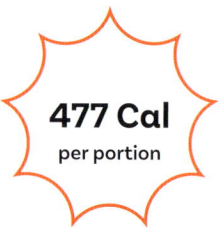
477 Cal per portion

Protein: 35.1g   **Fat: 11.1g**   **Carbs: 54.8g**

SERVES 4

I love using pork mince in fried rice recipes to add another dimension of flavour. It's sweet yet savoury and is packed full of protein, and veggies for nutrients. Usually leftover cooked rice is used in fried rice recipes, but if you're anything like me, you either forget or you never have any left. Using microwave rice and leaving it to cool helps to create this fried rice for a speedy quick fix.

Ingredients

2 × 250g packets of microwave long-grain rice
1 tsp sesame oil
500g lean pork mince
2 × 135g packets of frozen vegetables (peas, carrot, sweetcorn)
2 tsp chopped garlic
1 tsp chopped ginger
4 spring onions, sliced
35g runny honey
30g reduced-sugar ketchup
30ml light soy sauce
30ml dark soy sauce
2 tbsp oyster sauce
2 medium eggs, whisked
50ml water (if needed)

NOTE
To reheat, loosen with water, and you can always add a dash of soy sauce too.

Method

- Start by microwaving the packets of rice according to the packet instructions. Once cooked, pour onto a large baking tray and leave to cool.

- Meanwhile, heat a large wok over a high heat. Add the sesame oil and leave it for 30 seconds to get hot before adding the pork mince. Fry for 5-7 minutes, until almost cooked, leaving it undisturbed for a couple of minutes on each side before flipping to help the mince crisp up.

- Next, microwave the vegetable bags as per the packet instructions.

- Once the mince is crispy, add the garlic and ginger, along with half the spring onions. Mix well for 30 seconds, then add 20g of the honey, 15g of the ketchup, 20ml of the light soy sauce, 20ml of the dark soy sauce and a tablespoon of the oyster sauce. Leave over a medium heat for a couple of minutes to allow the pork to soak up the flavours.

- After a couple of minutes, add the cooked rice, stirring well to combine with the pork (if you want extra crispy rice, leave on a high heat for a couple of minutes without moving it around.

- Add the remaining honey (15g), ketchup (15g), light soy (10ml), dark soy (10ml) and tablespoon of oyster sauce. Mix well before making a small well in the centre. Pour in the whisked eggs, leaving for a minute to set before breaking up into chunks and scrambling them.

- Finally, add the cooked vegetables and loosen with the water, if needed, to help the ingredients combine. Serve with the remaining spring onions on top.

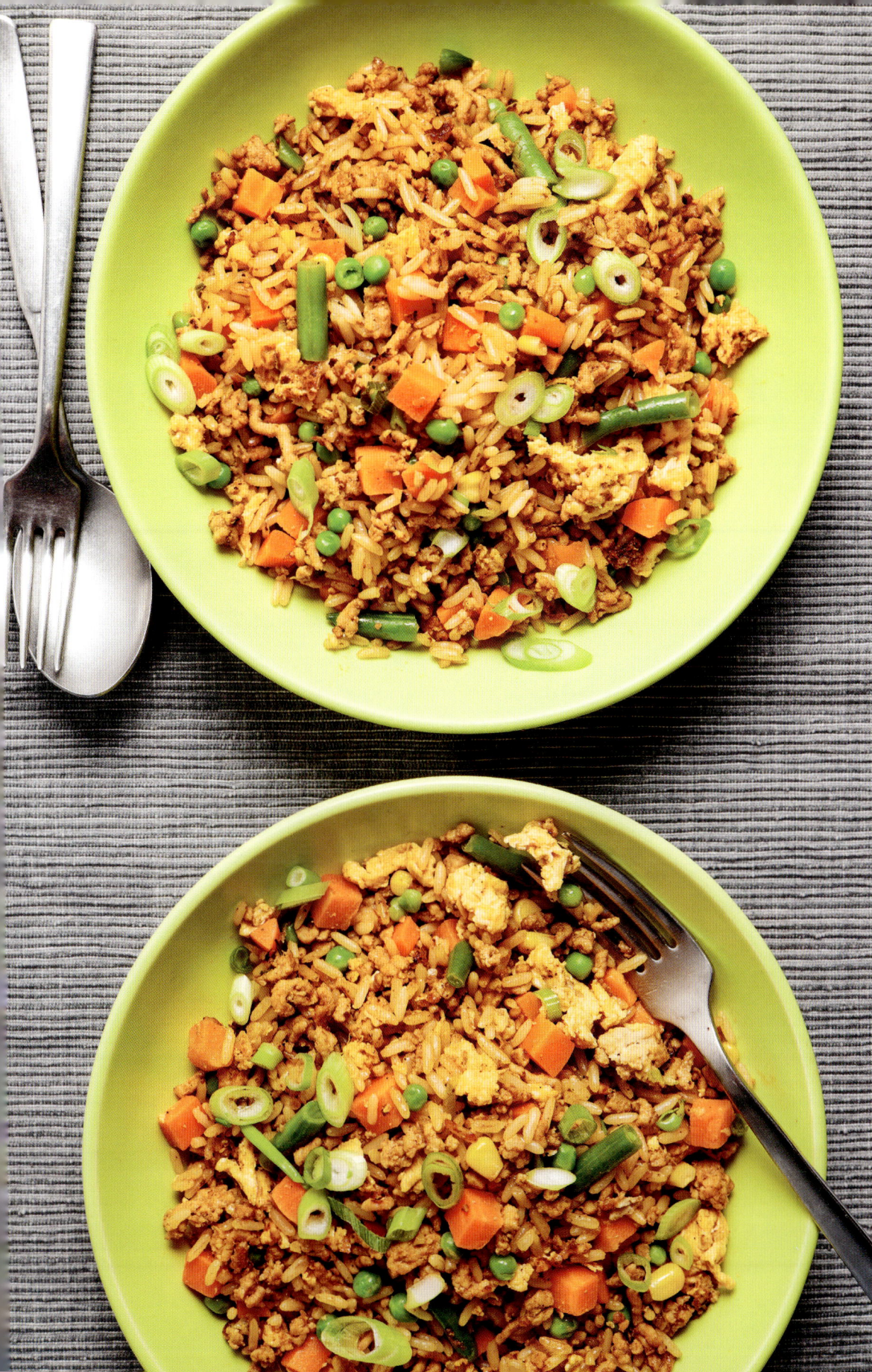

Bolognese Potato Bake

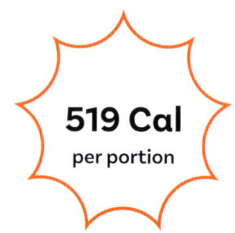

519 Cal per portion

| Protein: 42.5g | Fat: 16.7g | Carbs: 42.5g |

SERVES 4

My favourite meal of all time is a spaghetti bolognese, so it's no surprise I'm constantly on the hunt for different ways to use a bolognese sauce. For this recipe, it's paired with frozen crispy potatoes for added quickness, along with a homemade béchamel sauce and plenty of cheese for a serious comfort dinner fix.

Ingredients

300g frozen crispy potatoes
Olive oil spray
1 white onion, diced
1 small carrot, diced
400g lean beef mince
2 tsp chopped garlic
2 tsp Italian herb seasoning
1 tbsp Worcestershire sauce
1 tbsp tomato purée
1 × 400g tin of chopped tomatoes
150ml hot beef stock
100g reduced-fat cheddar, grated
Salt and pepper
A few sprigs of fresh parsley, chopped, to garnish

Béchamel sauce
20g light butter
20g plain flour
200ml semi-skimmed milk

Method

- Start by air frying the potatoes for 14 minutes at 190°C. Preheat the grill to high.

- Meanwhile, heat a large frying pan over a high heat. Spray with a few pumps of olive oil spray, add the diced onion and carrot and fry for 2 minutes, until softened.

- Add the mince and fry for 3–4 minutes, until almost browned.

- While the beef cooks, place the butter for the béchamel in a separate saucepan and melt over a low heat.

- Once the beef is almost browned, add the chopped garlic along with the Italian herb seasoning and fry for a further 30 seconds. Then add the Worcestershire sauce, tomato purée, chopped tomatoes and beef stock. Leave over a medium heat to simmer.

- Meanwhile, once the butter has melted, stir through the flour to form a roux (a thick paste). Gradually pour in the milk, whisking to combine. Keep stirring over a medium heat until a thick sauce has formed. Season with a pinch of salt and pepper before removing from the heat.

- Arrange the cooked potatoes on top of the beef mince, then pour over the béchamel sauce before topping with the cheddar.

- Pop the pan under the hot grill for 3–4 minutes until the cheese has melted.

- Serve with the fresh parsley scattered on top.

Oven To cook the potatoes in the oven, just follow the instructions on the packet.

Greek-Style Chicken Orzo

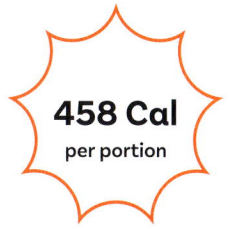

458 Cal per portion

`Protein: 41.5g` `Fat: 7.8g` `Carbs: 46.9g`

SERVES 4

I love using orzo in recipes where I fancy a 'lighter' pasta. In this recipe it is paired with juicy sliced chicken seasoned with Greek-inspired flavours, along with crumbled feta for a delicious dinner. Chicken thighs work well with this recipe and if you want to bulk it out further, you can add some fresh cherry tomatoes and diced courgette.

Ingredients

4 × 100g skinless chicken breasts, flattened
2 tsp smoked paprika
2 tsp oregano
3 tsp lemon juice
2 tsp chopped garlic
1 tbsp fat-free Greek yoghurt
240g dried orzo
Olive oil spray
1 large red pepper, diced
1 large red onion, diced
¼ tsp chilli flakes (optional)
½ tsp dried parsley
1 tbsp tomato purée
1 × 400g tin of chopped tomatoes
1 chicken stock cube, crumbled
100ml water
60g feta, crumbled
Salt and pepper

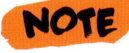

To make this veggie, use a vegetable stock cube and halloumi in place of the chicken.

Method

- Preheat the oven to 220ºC/200ºC fan.
- Start by putting the chicken breasts into a large bowl. Season with 1 teaspoon of the smoked paprika, 1 teaspoon of the oregano, 2 teaspoons of the lemon juice, 1 teaspoon of the chopped garlic, the Greek yoghurt and some salt and pepper. Place on a baking tray and bake in the oven for 16 minutes, until cooked through.
- Next, add the orzo to a large pan of boiling salted water and cook according to the packet instructions.
- Spray a large frying pan with olive oil spray. Sauté the red pepper and onion for a couple of minutes, until soft.
- Once soft, stir in the remaining teaspoon of garlic for 30 seconds, before adding the remaining smoked paprika, oregano and lemon juice, the chilli flakes, if using, the dried parsley and some salt and pepper to taste.
- Mix well, then add the tomato purée, chopped tomatoes, crumbled stock cube and water. Turn the heat down low to simmer.
- When the orzo is ready, drain and stir it into the tomato mix. Add half of the crumbled feta and stir through before removing from the heat.
- Slice the cooked chicken into strips.
- Serve the orzo with the chicken on top, along with the remaining crumbled feta.

Air Fryer Cook the chicken for 14 minutes at 190ºC.

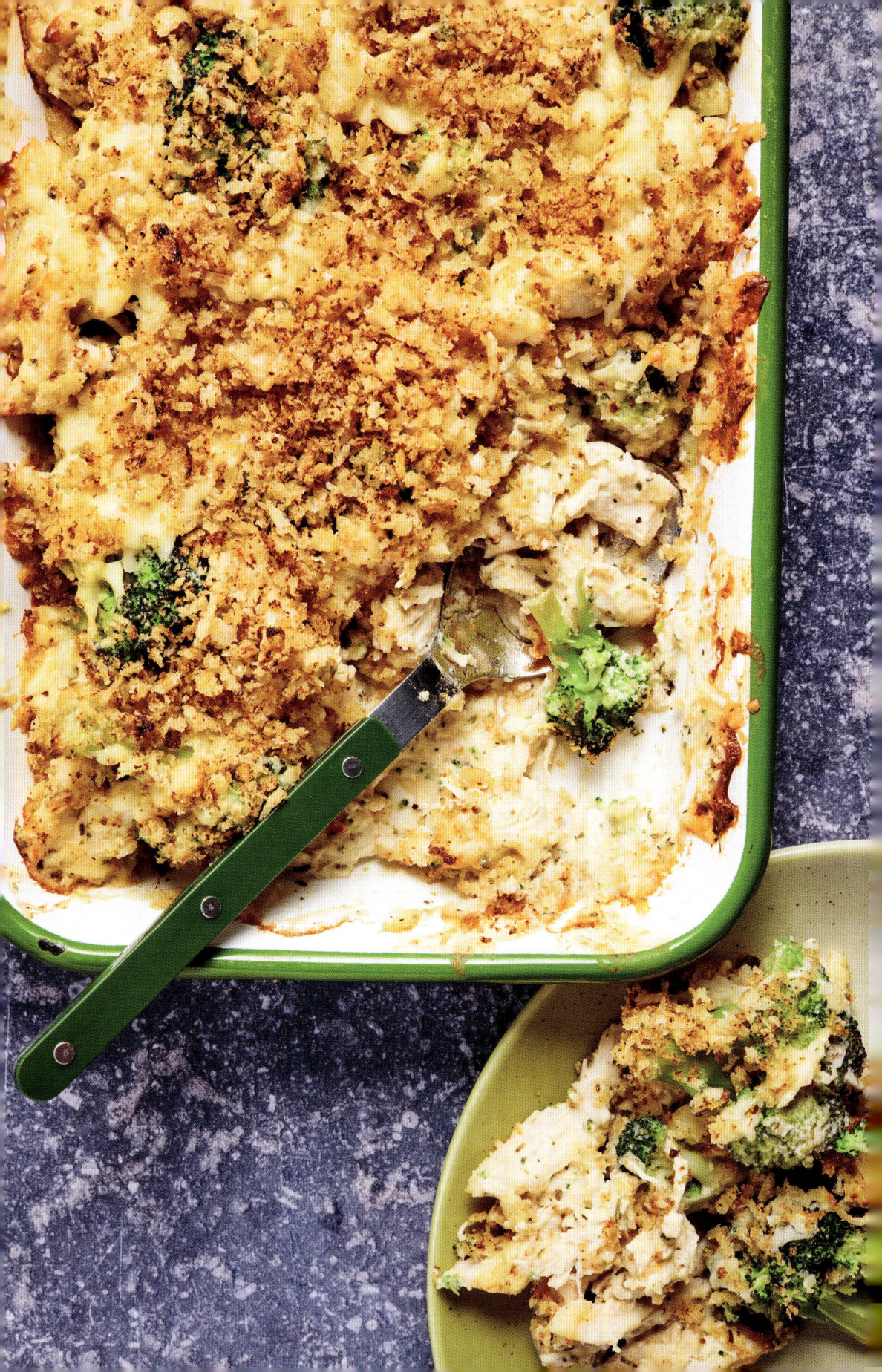

Garlic Crumb Chicken and Broccoli Bake

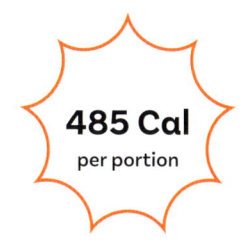

485 Cal per portion

| Protein: 61.2g | Fat: 17.6g | Carbs: 17.1g |

SERVES 3 (large portions)

This is one of those gorgeous comfort recipes for when you need a pick-me-up. It's packed full of flavour thanks to crunchy golden garlic breadcrumbs, a creamy garlic and herb shredded chicken and broccoli mix, and loads of cheddar and Parmesan. If you don't like broccoli you can swap it for cauliflower. This recipe makes three good-sized portions, but if you plan to have a carb source with it, such as crispy potatoes, it will serve four.

Ingredients

1 head of broccoli, chopped
10g light butter
1 tsp chopped garlic
25g panko breadcrumbs
400g cooked skinless chicken breast, shredded
1 tsp garlic granules
1 tsp onion granules
1 tsp mixed herbs
150g reduced-fat garlic and herb cream cheese (room temperature)
1 chicken stock cube, crumbled
50ml semi-skimmed milk
1 tsp cornflour
100g reduced-fat cheddar, grated
20g Parmesan, grated
Salt and pepper

Method

- Preheat the oven to 210°C/190°C fan.
- Cook the broccoli in a large pan of boiling water for 5 minutes. Once cooked, drain and leave to one side.
- Meanwhile, make the garlicky breadcrumbs by adding the butter to a hot pan over a medium heat. Once slightly melted, add the chopped garlic followed by the breadcrumbs. Cook for 5 minutes, tossing here and there to encourage browning all over.
- In a large bowl, combine the shredded chicken, garlic granules, onion granules and mixed herbs before seasoning with salt and pepper, then add the cream cheese, chicken stock cube, milk and cornflour. Mix well before stirring through half the cheese.
- Add the cooked broccoli to a large baking dish (about 25 × 25cm). Pour in the chicken mix and toss everything to combine.
- Top with the remaining cheddar before layering the crunchy breadcrumbs and Parmesan on top.
- Bake in the centre of the oven for 10 minutes, until the cheese has melted. Remove and serve.

Honey BBQ Sausages and Potatoes

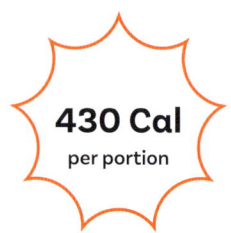

430 Cal per portion

Protein: 17.9g   **Fat: 16.1g**   **Carbs: 47g**

SERVES 4

There is nothing quite like the combination of barbecue flavours with pork sausage. This recipe is a traybake-style dinner but it is all done on the hob in a fraction of the time. If you want to up the protein in this recipe, you can use chicken or turkey sausages instead of the pork. I like to have this with a crispy salad but you can also pair it with some broccoli if you prefer.

Ingredients

750g baby potatoes, halved
Olive oil spray
8 reduced-fat pork sausages
1 red onion, cut into chunks
1 red pepper, cut into chunks
1 green pepper, cut into chunks
3 tsp barbecue seasoning
1 tsp smoked paprika
1 tsp chopped garlic
90g barbecue sauce
20g runny honey
1 tsp tomato purée
50ml water
40g ranch dressing (optional)
Salt and pepper
A few sprigs of fresh parsley, chopped, to garnish

Method

- Start by placing the potatoes in a large pan of boiling water and cook for 12–14 minutes, until tender when pierced with a fork.

- Meanwhile, spray a large frying pan with a few pumps of olive oil spray. Add the sausages and fry over a high heat for 8 minutes. Once browned, add the onion and peppers and fry for a further 2 minutes, until slightly softened.

- Once the veggies have softened, turn down the heat and add 2 teaspoons of the barbecue seasoning, the smoked paprika and chopped garlic, along with a pinch of salt and pepper.

- Mix well to combine before adding the barbecue sauce, honey, tomato purée and water. Stir until all of the ingredients are coated in the sauce and turn the heat down to low.

- Once the potatoes are cooked, drain and season them with salt, pepper and the remaining teaspoon of barbecue seasoning.

- Serve the cooked potatoes with the sausage and pepper mix on top. Drizzle over the ranch dressing, if using, and garnish with the fresh parsley.

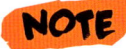

When reheating, add a tablespoon of water to the sauce to help loosen it. If your pan isn't large enough for the potatoes to cook in plenty of room, it's best to use two to allow them to cook quicker.

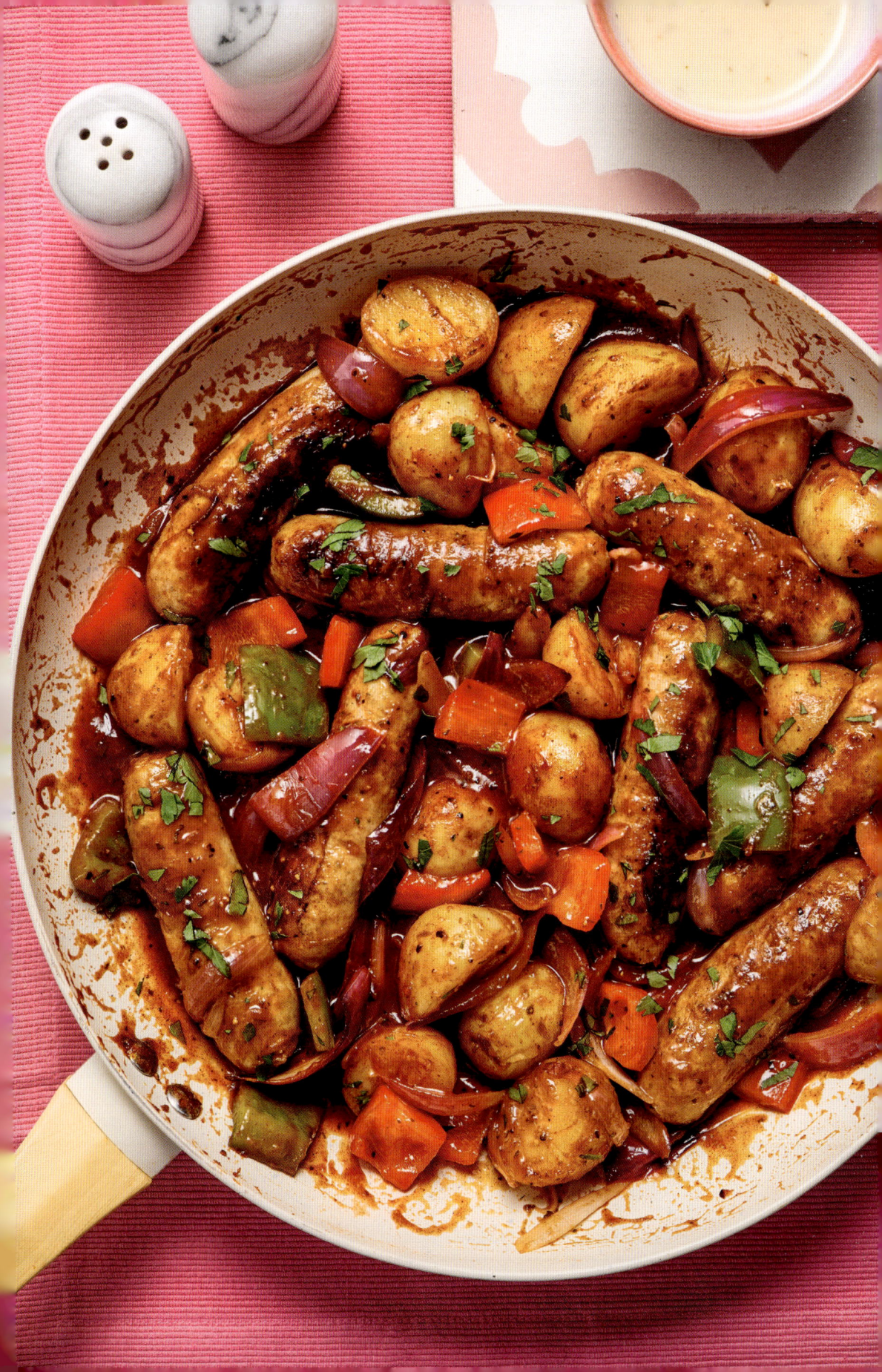

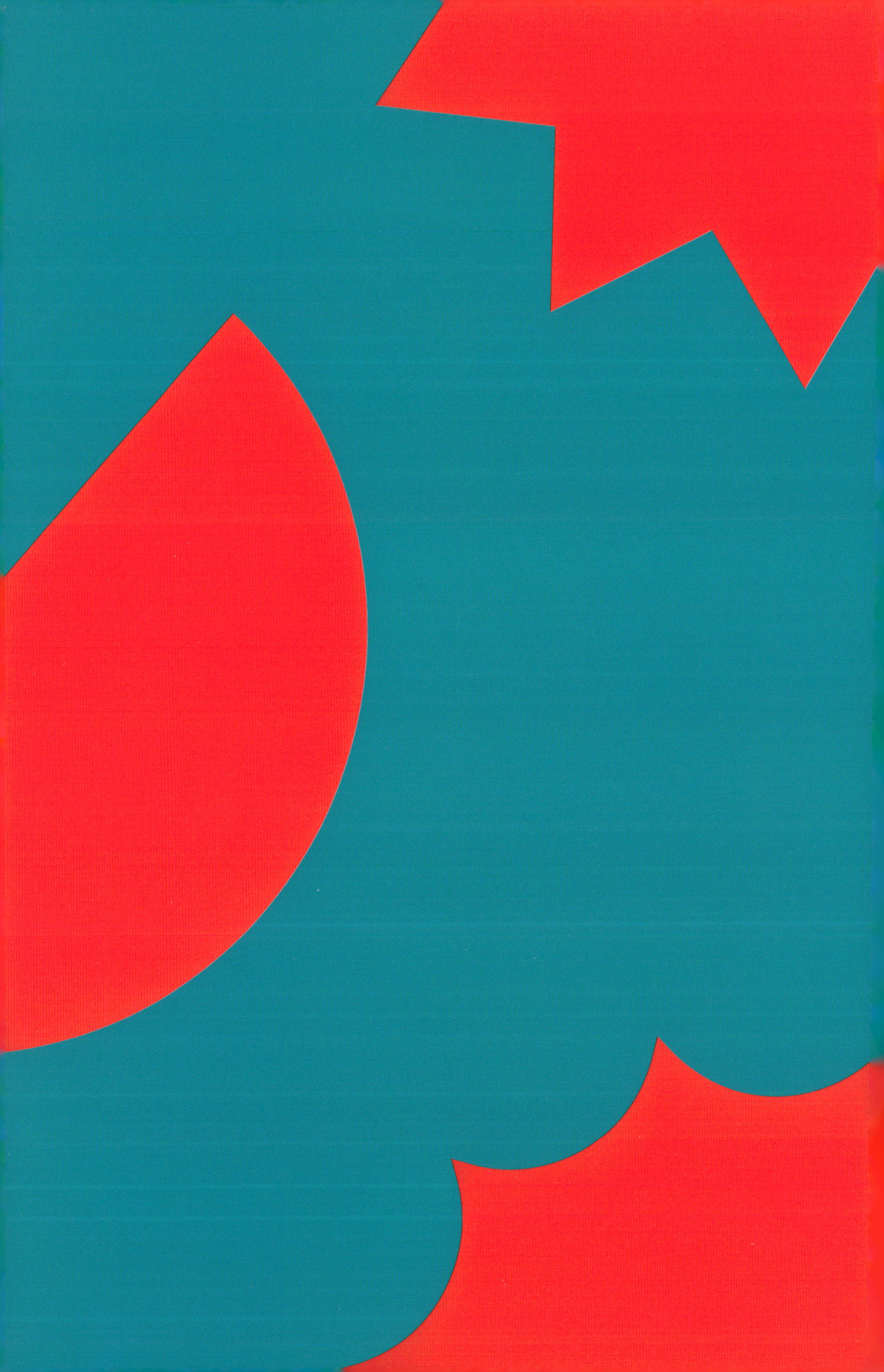

Five

DINNERS IN A JIFFY

Crunchy Garlic Butter Salmon Bites with Couscous

581 Cal per portion

Protein: 37.3g   Fat: 24.7g   Carbs: 46.2g

SERVES 2

When I say this recipe will knock your socks off, I mean it. If you don't like fish, sub the salmon for cubed chicken pieces. I love to serve this recipe with some pan-fried garlic and lemon broccoli.

Ingredients

5g light butter

1 tsp chopped garlic

30g panko breadcrumbs

2 salmon fillets (260g in total), skin removed and cut into 2.5cm cubes

1 tsp smoked paprika

1 tsp garlic granules

10g Parmesan, grated

1 small egg, whisked

Olive oil spray

1 × 110g packet of roasted vegetable couscous

Salt and pepper

2 sprigs of fresh parsley, chopped, to garnish

Sauce

20g light butter

1 tsp chopped garlic

1 tsp lemon juice

1 tsp chopped fresh parsley

Method

- Preheat the oven to 220°C/200°C fan.
- For the salmon, start by adding the butter to a small frying pan. Over a high heat, leave the butter to melt, then add the chopped garlic and breadcrumbs. Toast for around a minute and a half until slightly golden.
- While the breadcrumbs cook, season the salmon all over with the smoked paprika and garlic granules along with a pinch of salt and pepper.
- Once the breadcrumbs are done, transfer to a plate along with the grated Parmesan, tossing to combine.
- Dip each piece of salmon into the whisked egg, shaking off any excess, before dipping into the breadcrumbs.
- Spray a large baking tray with a few pumps of olive oil spray and transfer each salmon bite to the tray. Bake in the oven for 12 minutes.
- When there are 6 minutes remaining on the salmon, heat a small pan over a low heat. Add all of the sauce ingredients and leave to simmer.
- Next, make the couscous according to the packet instructions.
- Transfer the couscous to a bowl.
- Once the salmon is cooked, pile the salmon bites in the centre of the couscous. Drizzle over the garlic butter sauce and garnish with the fresh parsley.

Air Fryer Air fry the salmon bites at 180°C for 8–10 minutes, depending on the thickness of the salmon.

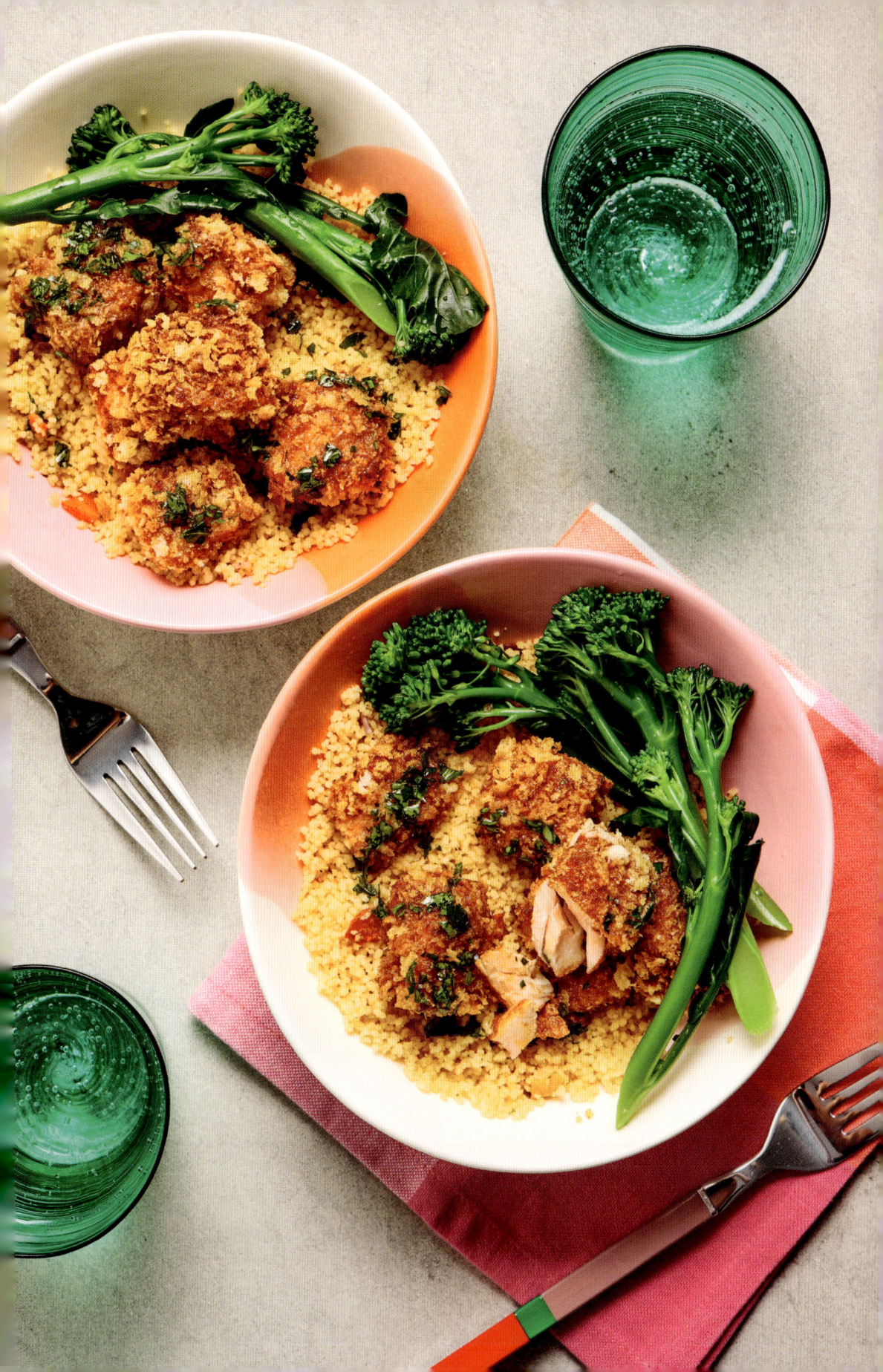

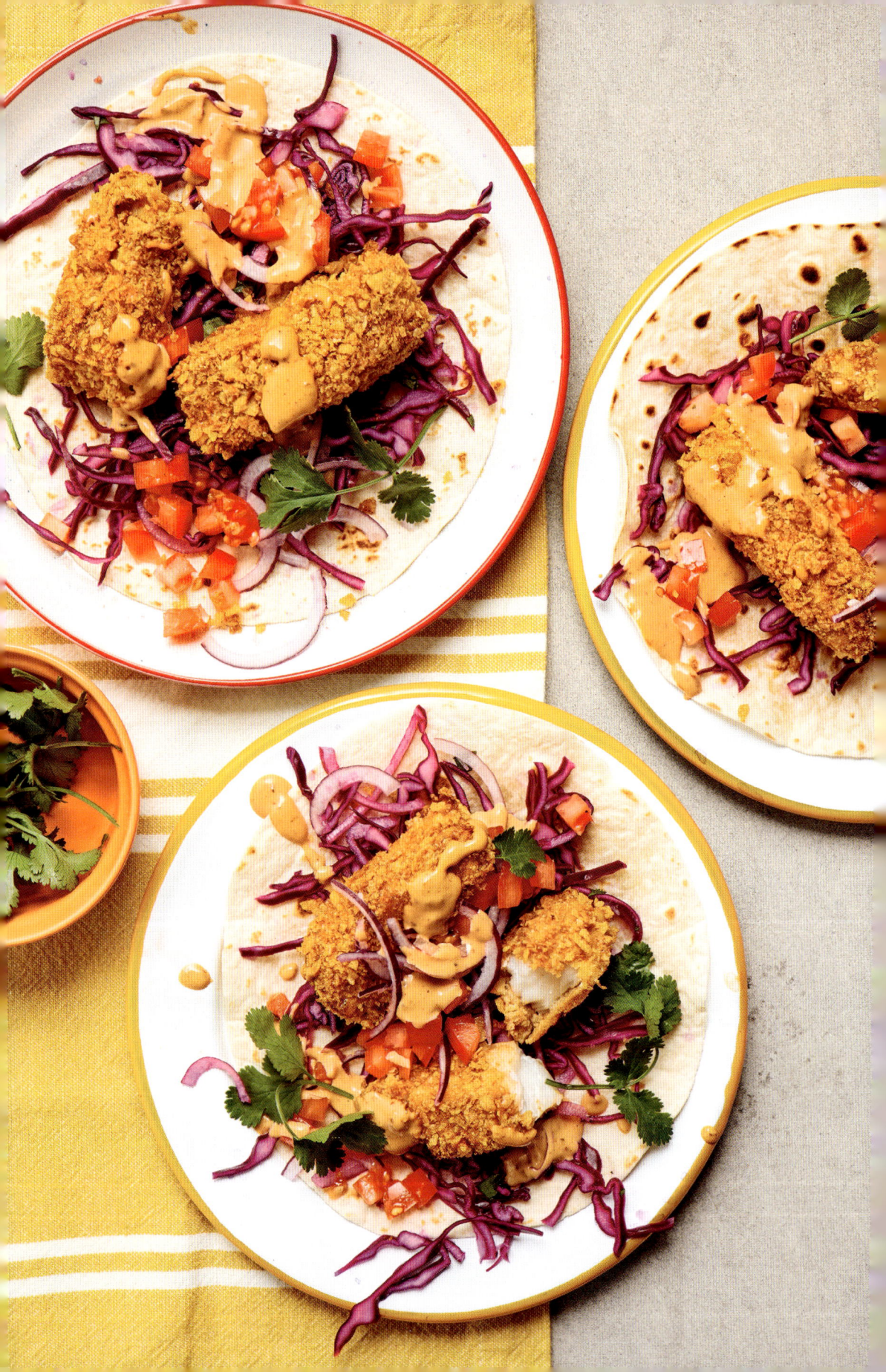

Baja-Style Fish Tacos

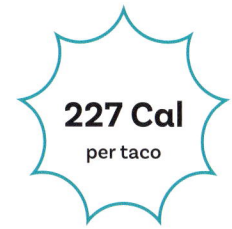

227 Cal per taco

Protein: 19.2g   Fat: 3.9g   Carbs: 21.8g

SERVES 2

These tacos are exploding with flavour. Traditionally, they are battered, but for a lighter bite this recipe calls for crushed cornflakes. If you want to bulk them out further, you can add some crumbled feta, smashed avocado or a tomato salsa.

Ingredients

2 × 130g cod fillets
1 tsp garlic granules
1 tsp ground cumin
½ tsp paprika
1 medium egg, whisked
30g cornflakes, finely crushed
¼ head of red cabbage, thinly sliced
1 red onion, sliced
4 sprigs of fresh coriander, chopped
100ml distilled white vinegar
1 tbsp lime juice
4 white mini tortilla wraps
2 salad tomatoes, diced

Chipotle sauce
50g lighter than light mayonnaise
1 tsp chipotle paste
1 tsp lime juice
½ tsp garlic granules
Pinch of salt

Method

- Start by patting the fish fillets dry. Season all over with the garlic granules, cumin and paprika. Slice each fillet into four fish-finger shapes.
- Dip each fish finger into the egg, shaking off any excess before dipping into the cornflakes. Press the cornflakes down carefully to stick them to the fish.
- Place the fish directly in the air fryer and cook for 14 minutes at 180°C.
- While the fish cooks, first put the red cabbage, red onion and three quarters of the coriander into a jar along with the distilled white vinegar. Pour in the lime juice and fill with 250ml water. Close the lid and give it a good shake. Set to one side.
- Meanwhile, make up the chipotle sauce by mixing all the ingredients together, then set to one side.
- Place each tortilla wrap in a large dry frying pan over a high heat and toast for 45–60 seconds on each side until slightly crispy.
- Top each wrap with some pickled cabbage and crispy fish, followed by the chipotle sauce, then finish with the diced tomatoes and remaining coriander.

Oven Preheat the oven to 220°C/200°C fan and cook the fish fingers for 16 minutes.

Lemon Pepper Chicken

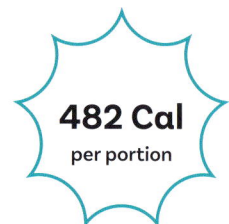

482 Cal per portion

| Protein: 40.7g | Fat: 9.3g | Carbs: 56g |

SERVES 2

Serve a flavoursome dinner with this tasty recipe of sweet, tangy and tender bites of chicken and rice. You can use this recipe with chicken thighs or even fish if you fancy a change.

Ingredients

1 × 125g packet of boil-in-the-bag rice

250g skinless chicken breast, cut into 2.5cm cubes

1 tsp chopped garlic

1 tsp onion granules

¼ tsp paprika

Pinch of salt

½ tsp cracked black pepper

Juice of ½ small lemon

Olive oil spray

A few sprigs of fresh parsley, to garnish

Sauce

1 tsp chopped garlic

20g light butter

Juice of ½ small lemon

Zest of 1 lemon

1 tbsp light soy sauce

10g runny honey

¼ tsp red chilli flakes (optional)

Salt and pepper

Method

- Start by cooking the rice according to the packet instructions.
- Add the cubed chicken to a bowl with the chopped garlic, onion granules, paprika, salt, black pepper and lemon juice. Give it a good stir.
- Next, heat a large frying pan over a medium-high heat. Spray with a few pumps of olive oil spray, add the chicken to the pan and fry for around 8 minutes, until cooked through, then remove from the pan.
- Meanwhile, add all of the sauce ingredients to a bowl and stir to combine.
- When there are only a few minutes remaining on the rice, add the sauce ingredients to the frying pan and leave over a medium heat to thicken. Once thickened, return the chicken to the pan and toss to combine.
- Serve the cooked chicken over the rice and garnish with the fresh parsley.

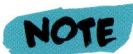

This recipe will store in the fridge for up to 3 days. Loosen with a splash of water when reheating.

Halloumi Souvlaki Flatbreads

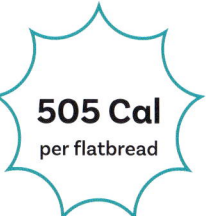

505 Cal per flatbread

Protein: 29.7g   Fat: 20.6g   Carbs: 49.4g

SERVES 2

Pan-fried halloumi is always a go-to for me when we're having a meat-free dinner. It pairs perfectly with Greek-inspired flavours in a fluffy flatbread and an aubergine, onion and tomato mix that's tossed with balsamic glaze. If you have the calories to spare, why not throw in some fries?

Ingredients

Olive oil spray
100g aubergine, thinly sliced widthways
175g reduced-fat halloumi, cut into bite-sized cubes
1 tsp oregano
½ tsp dried thyme
¼ tsp paprika
1 tsp lemon juice
1 tsp chopped garlic
2 Greek-style flatbreads
1 red onion, sliced
2 large tomatoes, diced
1 tbsp balsamic glaze
30g tzatziki dip

Method

- Spray a medium frying pan with olive oil spray and set over a medium-high heat. Add the aubergine slices, ensuring they are not overlapping and that there is space surrounding each piece. Cook for around 8 minutes, turning them throughout the cooking time, until they are almost browned on each side and their centres feel slightly squidgy.
- Meanwhile, put the halloumi into a bowl. Season with half the oregano, the dried thyme, paprika, lemon juice and garlic. Mix well to combine.
- Spray a separate clean frying pan with olive oil spray. Add the halloumi and cook for 1–2 minutes before flipping and cooking for the same amount of time on the other side or until golden. Once cooked, remove from the heat.
- Grill the flatbreads according to the packet instructions.
- Once the aubergine is cooked, add the sliced red onion and diced tomatoes. Fry for a further minute before adding in the balsamic glaze, 2 tablespoons of water and the remaining half teaspoon of oregano.
- Put the vegetable mix along one half of each flatbread and top with the halloumi, followed by the tzatziki. Fold over the other half of the flatbread to serve.

Chilli Garlic Prawn Linguine

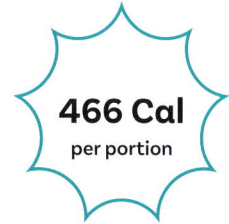
466 Cal per portion

| Protein: 27.9g | Fat: 10g | Carbs: 63.6g |

SERVES 2

This is one of those speedy dinners that really feels like a dining experience at home. Prawns are tossed with linguine in a simple chilli, onion and garlic sauce and finished with crispy chorizo pieces to add a touch of smokiness to the dish.

Ingredients

140g dried linguine
40g chorizo, diced
1 white onion, diced
1 red chilli, chopped
2 tsp chopped garlic
120g cherry tomatoes, halved
1 tbsp tomato purée
1 tsp smoked paprika
165g raw peeled king prawns
1 tbsp lemon juice
1 tbsp (20g) reduced-fat crème fraîche
4 sprigs of fresh parsley, chopped
1 tsp chilli flakes (optional)
Salt and pepper

Method

- Start by cooking the linguine in a large pan of boiling salted water according to the packet instructions. Once cooked, drain, reserving a ladleful of the water.
- Add the diced chorizo to a frying pan and fry for 2–3 minutes, until crispy. Remove from the pan, leaving the oils behind, and set to one side.
- Add the onion, chilli and garlic to the same pan and sauté for 2 minutes or until softened.
- Add the tomatoes and cook for around 4 minutes, until they have softened.
- Once the tomatoes are soft, add the tomato purée and smoked paprika and season with a good pinch of salt and pepper.
- Add the prawns to the same pan, cooking for a couple of minutes until they are fully pink.
- Add the lemon juice, crème fraîche, the ladleful of reserved pasta water and half of the chopped parsley. Give the sauce a quick stir before adding the linguine.
- Remove from the heat and ensure everything is tossed well.
- Serve with the crispy chorizo pieces on top, along with the remaining parsley and the chilli flakes, if using.

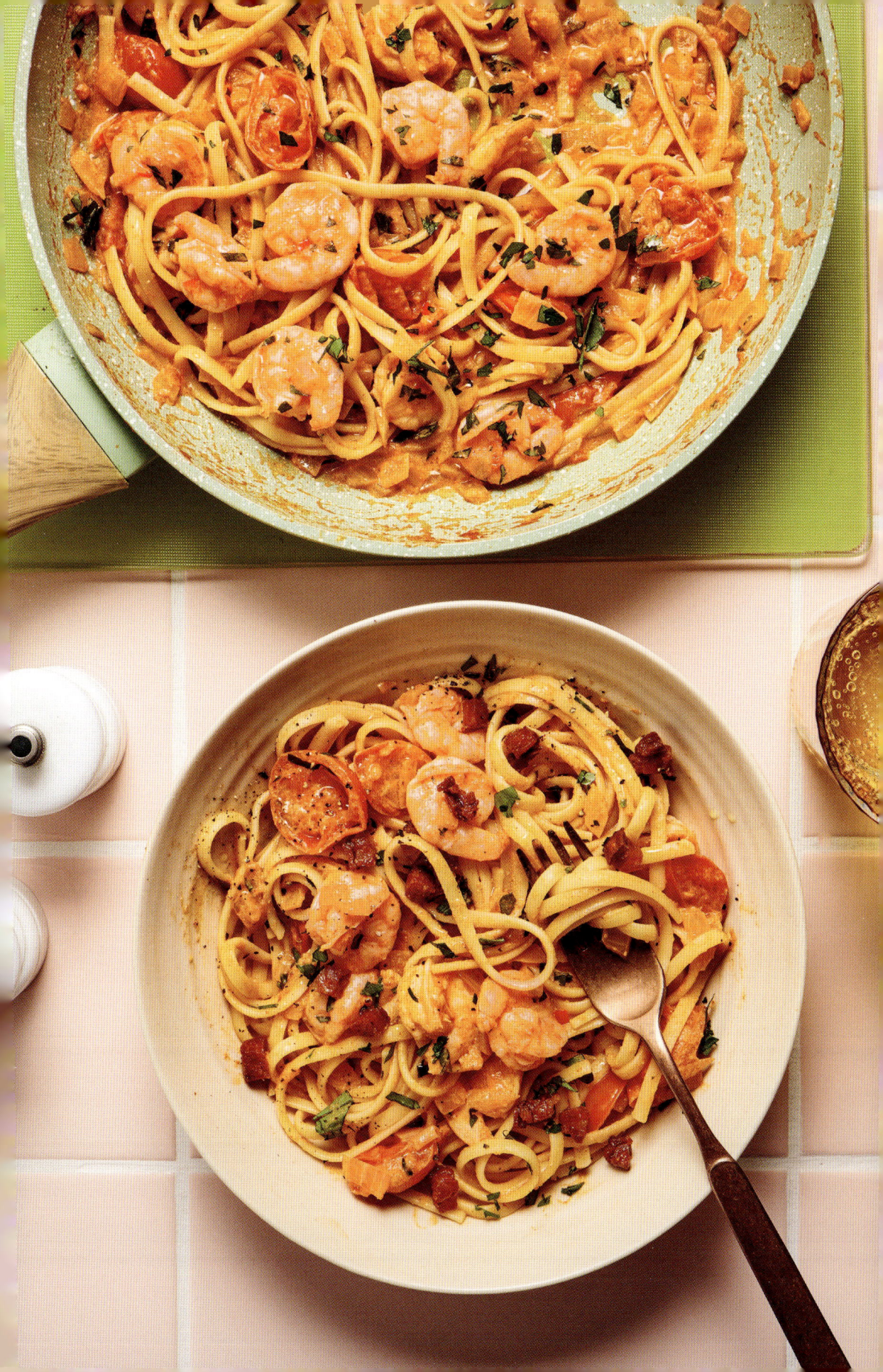

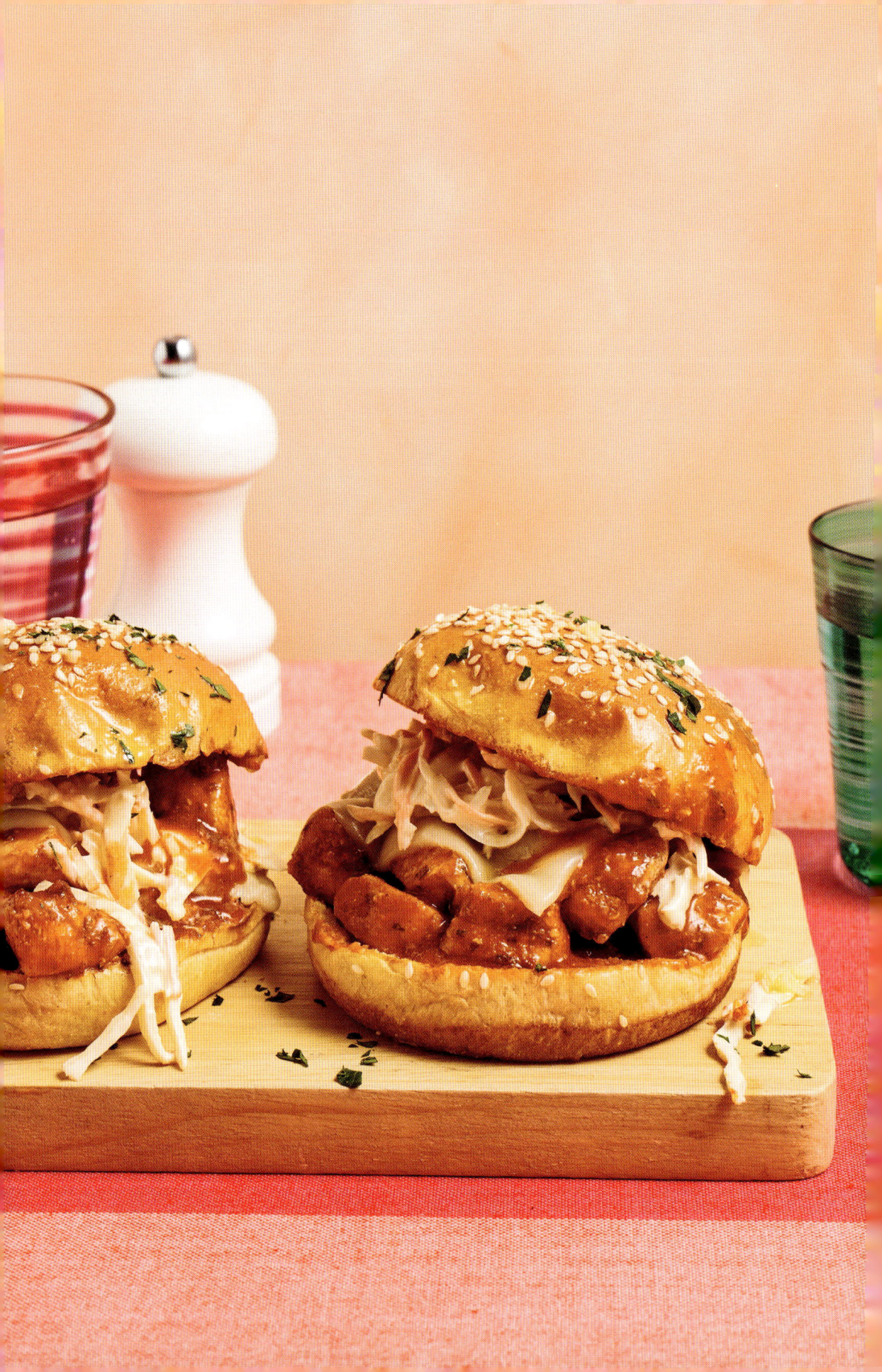

Spicy Chicken Sliders

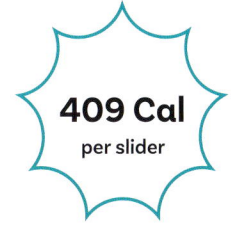

409 Cal per slider

`Protein: 39.9g`   `Fat: 13.5g`   `Carbs: 31.5g`

MAKES 4

These spicy sliders are the perfect balance of heat and cheesiness. I love to brush the garlic butter over the buns once they're baked rather than before, as this makes sure you get the burst of aromatic garlic butter to sink your teeth into before the buffalo flavours hit underneath. To bulk these sliders out further, you could add some red pepper or coleslaw.

Ingredients

400g skinless chicken breast, cut into 2.5cm cubes
1 tsp smoked paprika
1 tsp garlic granules
½ tsp onion granules
1 tsp dried oregano
4 brioche buns
4 mozzarella slices (the thin slices from a packet; 25g each)
20g light butter
50ml buffalo sauce
1 tbsp hot water
1 tsp chopped garlic
A couple of sprigs of fresh parsley, chopped

Method

- Preheat the oven to 210°C/190°C and heat a large frying pan over a medium-high heat.
- Add the chicken to a bowl, then season with the smoked paprika, garlic granules, onion granules and oregano. Rub the seasonings in thoroughly before transferring to the pan. Fry for 7-8 minutes, until cooked through.
- While the chicken cooks, slice the brioche buns in half. Toast each bottom bun until lightly golden. Transfer to a baking tray and then top with the cheese slices.
- Once the chicken has cooked, add half the butter to the pan and leave to melt, then add the buffalo sauce and water and mix well.
- Remove from the heat and top the bottom buns with the chicken. Cover with the top half of the bun and place in the oven for 5 minutes, until the cheese has melted.
- While the sliders are in the oven, put the remaining butter and the chopped garlic into a microwavable bowl. Blast for 10-15 seconds on medium until the butter has melted. Mix with a spoon.
- Remove the sliders from the oven and brush the tops of the buns with the garlic butter, then scatter over the parsley.

Thai Sweet Chilli Chicken Tenders

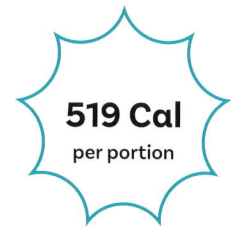

519 Cal per portion

Protein: 42.8g   Fat: 10.4g   Carbs: 61.45g

SERVES 2

Sometimes you just need chicken and chips for your tea. Here we've got crispy chicken tenders that are baked and tossed with a sweet chilli sauce and served along with sweet potato fries. If you want to save even more time, you can omit the coating step on the chicken.

Ingredients

150g frozen sweet potato fries
300g chicken breast mini fillets
1 tsp ground ginger
1 tsp garlic granules
½ tsp paprika
1 small egg, whisked
45g cornflakes, crushed
Olive oil spray
70g reduced-sugar Thai sweet chilli sauce
10ml light soy sauce
1 tsp sriracha sauce
10g runny honey
2 sprigs of fresh parsley, chopped
Salt and pepper

Method

- Start by preheating the oven to 240°C/220°C fan.
- Put the sweet potato fries into a large baking tray, ensuring they are not overlapping. Cook according to the packet instructions.
- Next, season the chicken all over with the ginger, garlic and paprika, along with a pinch of salt and pepper. Rub the seasonings into the chicken thoroughly.
- Dip each mini fillet into the egg, shaking off any excess, then dip them into the cornflakes. Press the cornflakes into the chicken to stick them down before transferring the fillets to a baking tray sprayed with oil.
- Bake the chicken for 15 minutes.
- Meanwhile, make up the sauce by combining the sweet chilli sauce, soy sauce, sriracha and honey. When there are a few minutes remaining on the chicken, pour the sauce into a pan and place over a low heat.
- Once the chicken is cooked, transfer it to a big bowl. Pour over the sauce and toss to combine.
- Serve the chicken scattered with the parsley and with the sweet potato fries alongside.

Air Fryer Cook the sweet potato fries according to the packet instructions. Cook the chicken at 200°C for 12 minutes.

Cajun Garlic Parmesan Chicken Skewers

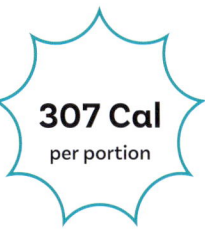

307 Cal per portion

| Protein: 44.4g | Fat: 11.8g | Carbs: 5.7g |

SERVES 2

AF

For all my garlic lovers, this one's for you. For a complete dinner, serve over a packet of Mexican rice or have with some frozen wedges.

Ingredients

300g skinless chicken breast, cut into 2.5cm cubes
2 tsp Cajun seasoning
½ tsp garlic granules
15g lighter than light mayonnaise
2 tsp lemon juice
Olive oil spray
15g light butter
1 tsp chopped garlic
10g Parmesan, grated
2 sprigs of fresh parsley, chopped

Method

- Start by removing any racks from the air fryer drawer and preheating it to 200ºC.
- Put the chicken into a bowl and add the Cajun seasoning, garlic granules, mayo and a teaspoon of the lemon juice. Mix well until combined.
- Thread the chicken pieces onto metal skewers, ensuring there is no space between the chicken pieces. If you have wooden skewers, make sure to soak them in water for 30 minutes prior to cooking to prevent them from burning.
- Spray the air fryer basket with olive oil spray and transfer the skewers to the drawer (if your basket isn't large enough for the skewers, you can just cook the chicken without them). Cook for 12 minutes, carefully turning partway through.
- While the chicken cooks, put the butter and garlic into a microwavable bowl. Blast for 15 seconds on medium, until the butter has melted. Stir through the Parmesan, the remaining teaspoon of lemon juice and three quarters of the parsley.
- When there are 5 minutes remaining of the chicken cooking time, baste the skewers with the juices in the air fryer basket, followed by three quarters of the garlic Parmesan sauce. Return to the basket for the remaining cooking time.
- Once the chicken is cooked and ready to serve, use the remaining sauce to brush over the skewers and sprinkle with the remaining parsley.

Oven You can cook these skewers in the oven by placing them on a baking tray and repeating the steps above. Bake for 16-18 minutes at 220ºC/200ºC fan.

Chipotle Chicken Fajitas

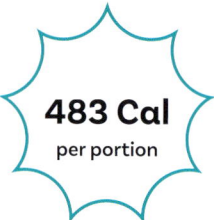

483 Cal per portion

Protein: 39.1g **Fat: 14.6g** **Carbs: 44.5g**

SERVES 2
(makes 4 mini wraps)

This is one of my ultimate quick and easy dinners that goes all the way back to my uni days and for good reason . . . It is packed full of flavour. You can swap the sour cream for Greek yoghurt, use half-fat cheddar, add avocado or make the fajitas veggie using halloumi – they are completely customisable to your fiesta. Feel free to make the filling ahead of time – it will keep in the fridge for a few days.

Ingredients

Olive oil spray

200g skinless chicken breast, cut into thin strips

1 heaped tbsp fajita seasoning

1 tbsp lime juice

1 tsp chipotle paste

1 small red pepper, sliced

1 small yellow pepper, sliced

1 small red onion, sliced

40g Mexican cheddar, grated

4 mini tortilla wraps

20g reduced-fat sour cream

2 tbsp tomato salsa

A few sprigs of fresh coriander, chopped

Method

- Start by spraying a large frying pan with olive oil spray and placing over a medium-high heat.
- While the pan heats, put the chicken, fajita seasoning, lime juice and chipotle paste into a mixing bowl. Mix well to combine, then add to the pan and fry for 4 minutes, until the chicken is part-cooked.
- Add the red and yellow pepper along with the red onion. Continue to fry for another 5 minutes until the chicken is cooked through and the veggies have softened, moving the chicken and veg around the pan continuously.
- Once the chicken is fully cooked, turn down the heat and stir through the cheddar.
- Place the wraps in the microwave and blast on medium for 20 seconds until slightly warm.
- Top each wrap with the chicken and veg. Divide the sour cream and tomato salsa equally between the wraps and scatter over the coriander.

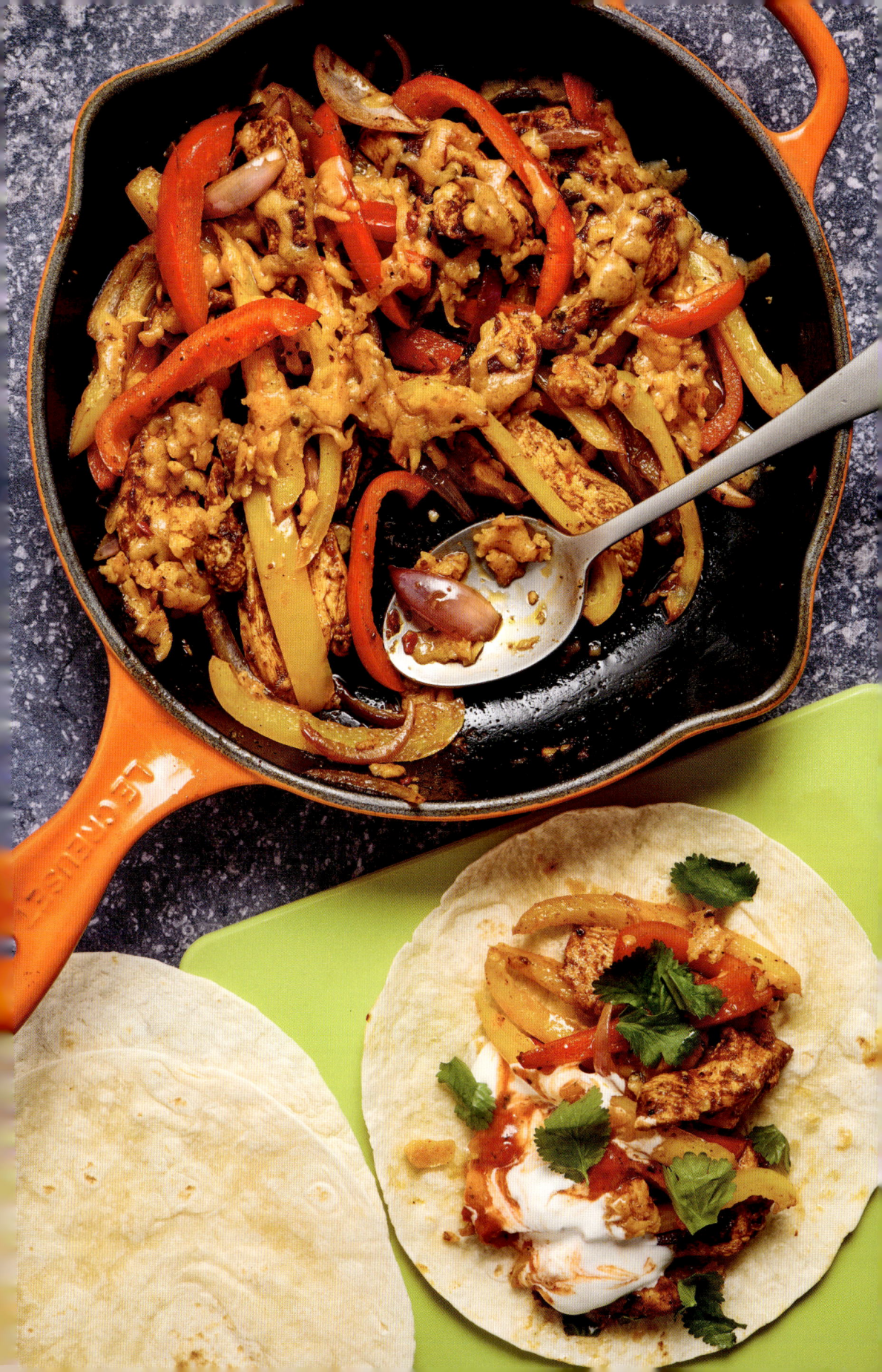

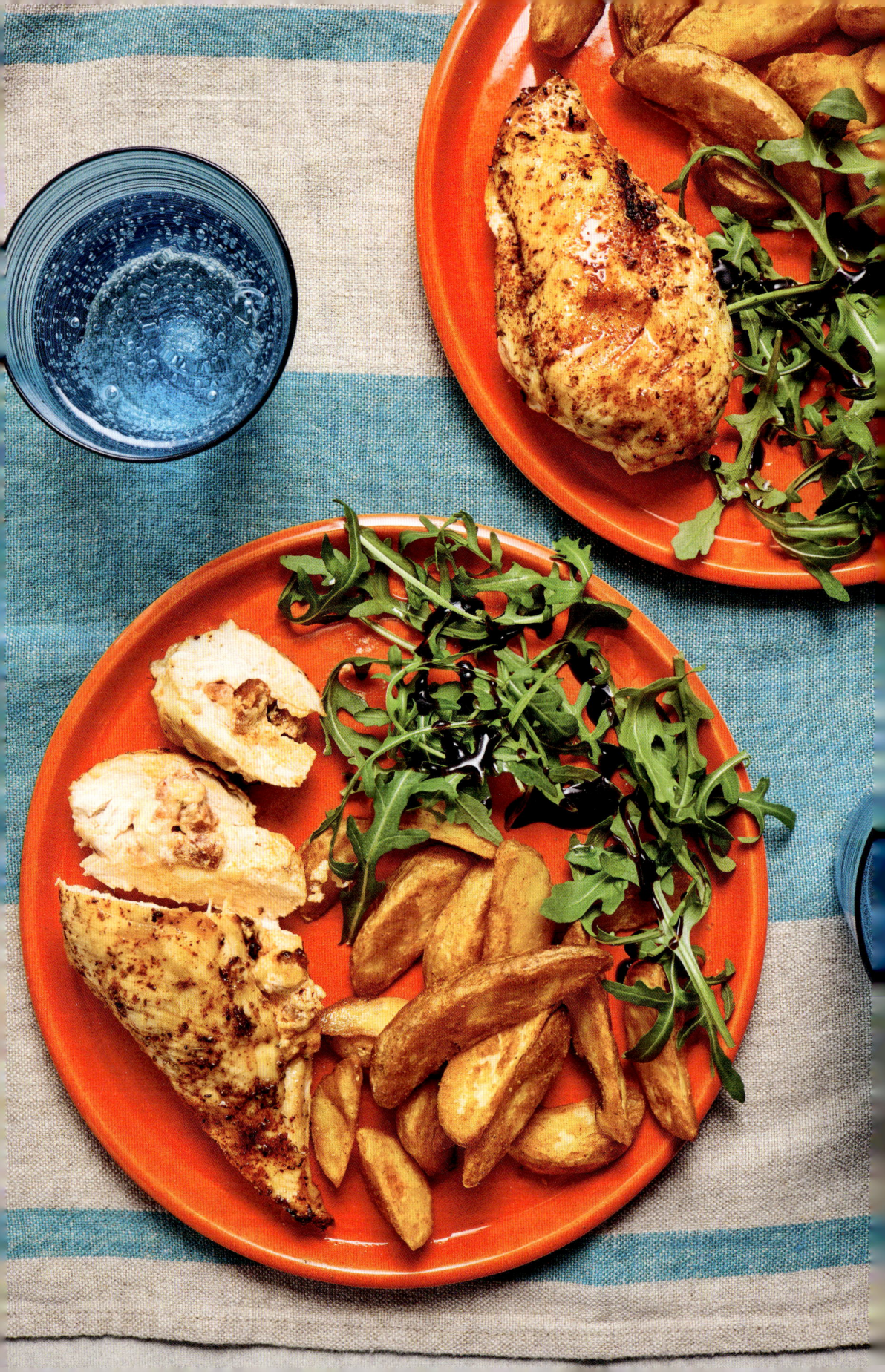

Sticky Chorizo Stuffed Chicken

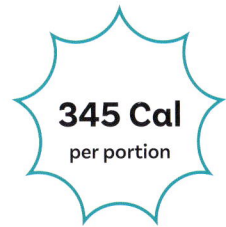

345 Cal per portion

| Protein: 48.4g | Fat: 12.8g | Carbs: 8.4g |

SERVES 2

This is one of those effortless dinners that tastes absolutely banging. Chicken breasts are stuffed with a mix of chorizo, mozzarella and cream cheese and brushed with honey to create a sticky surface. I like to pair these with baby potatoes, frozen wedges, a balsamic-glazed salad or some Tenderstem broccoli.

Ingredients

30g chorizo, finely diced
20g mozzarella, grated
20g light cream cheese
2 × 140g skinless chicken breasts
½ tsp oregano
½ tsp smoked paprika
15g runny honey

Method

- Preheat the air fryer to 195°C.
- Next, in a bowl, combine the diced chorizo, grated mozzarella and cream cheese.
- Prepare the chicken by slicing horizontally into the thickest part of the breasts, ensuring you do not slice all the way through.
- Stuff the chorizo cheese mixture into the flap of the chicken. Use your fingers to ensure the filling is pushed inside before closing the flap.
- Season the chicken with the oregano and smoked paprika, rubbing them over the top of each breast. Transfer the chicken to the air fryer basket and cook for 15 minutes. When there are 5 minutes remaining on the time, brush over half of the honey and return for the remaining time.
- Once cooked, remove from the air fryer and brush over the remaining honey to serve.

Oven Preheat the oven to 215°C/195°C fan and cook the chicken breasts for 20 minutes. Try to use chicken breasts that are not too thick and are long in length to help the cooking time.

Chicken, Bacon and Mozzarella Pasta

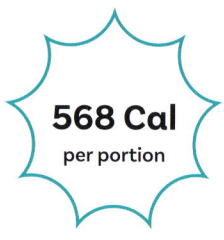

Protein: 46.8 **Fat: 18.2g** **Carbs: 48.1g**

SERVES 2

My social media followers went wild for this pasta dish and, truly, once you try it you will understand why. I like to serve this with some lightly steamed Tenderstem broccoli.

Ingredients

200g skinless chicken breast fillet, butterflied (or 2 thin 100g breasts)

2 tsp smoked paprika

1½ tsp garlic granules

2 tsp Italian herb seasoning

120g dried tagliatelle

Olive oil spray

2 rashers of streaky bacon, cut into strips

1 tbsp white wine vinegar

1 tsp chopped garlic

150ml reduced-fat single cream alternative (I use Elmlea)

40g mozzarella, grated

Salt and pepper

A few sprigs of fresh parsley, chopped, to garnish

NOTE

If you like super-crispy bacon, cook it under the grill for a couple of minutes instead of in the frying pan.

Method

- Preheat the oven to 220°C/200°C fan.

- Season the chicken with 1 teaspoon of the smoked paprika, 1 teaspoon of the garlic granules, 1 teaspoon of the Italian herb seasoning and some salt and pepper. Place on a non-stick baking tray and cook for 10 minutes.

- Meanwhile, cook the pasta in a large pan of salted water according to the packet instructions. Once cooked, drain the water into a jug, rinse the pasta under cold water and set to one side.

- Next, spray a frying pan with a few pumps of olive oil spray and fry the bacon strips over a high heat for 3-4 minutes until browned (or see the note below). Remove from the pan and set to one side.

- Return the pan to a medium heat, pour in the white wine vinegar to deglaze the bottom, scraping up any brown bits, then add the chopped garlic. Stir for 30 seconds, then add the cream, along with the remaining teaspoon of smoked paprika, ½ teaspoon of garlic granules and teaspoon of Italian herb seasoning. Leave to thicken for a few minutes.

- When the sauce has thickened, spoon a tablespoon over the chicken breasts and top with half the mozzarella. Place the tray back in the oven for 2 minutes.

- Meanwhile, add 50ml of the pasta water to the sauce along with the remaining mozzarella. Mix well until melted, then add the pasta to the sauce to heat through.

- Serve the cooked pasta with a chicken breast on top, along with the bacon strips, and garnished with fresh parsley.

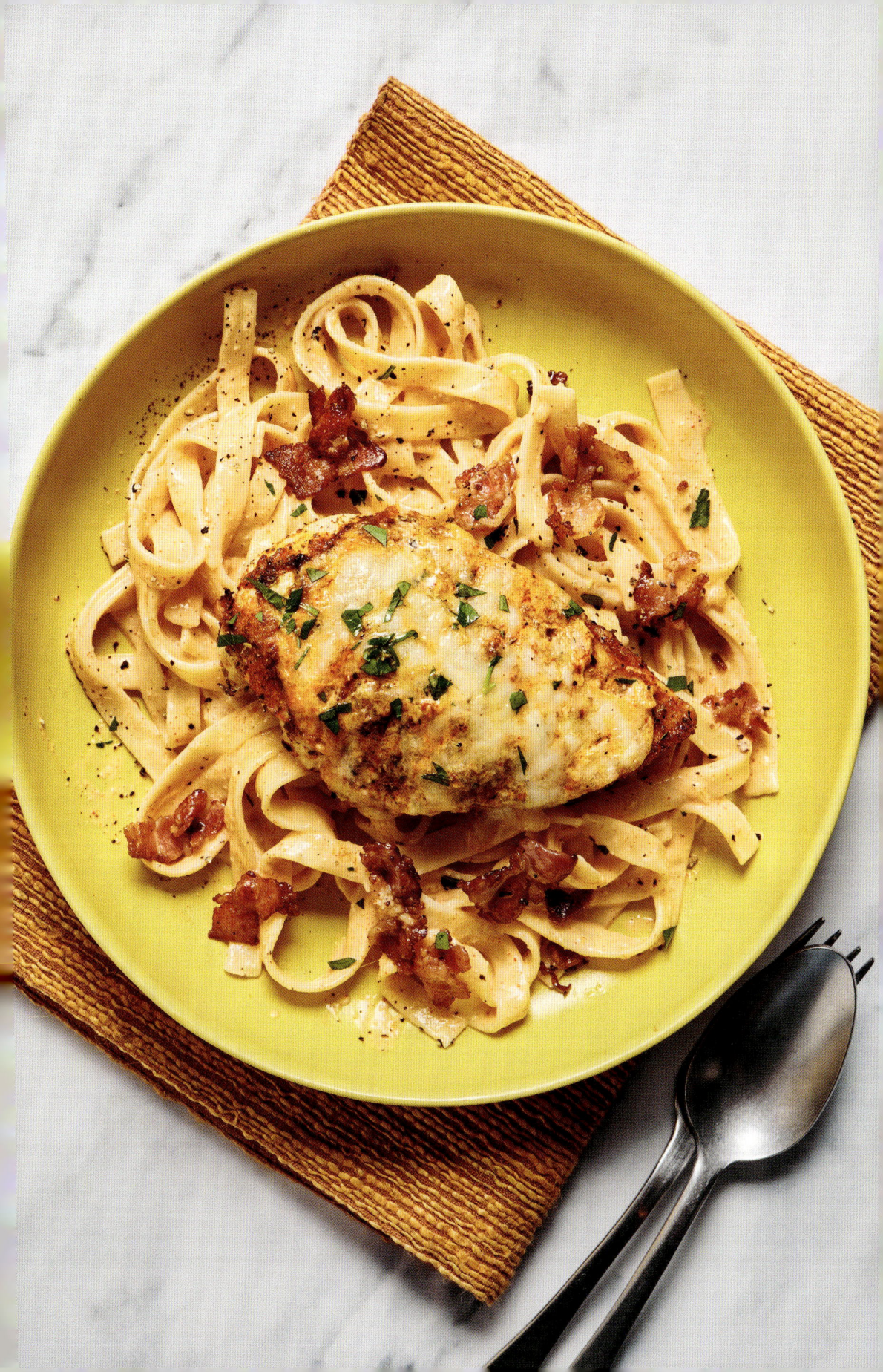

Bacon Cheeseburger Pasta

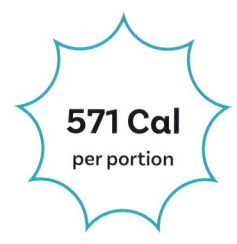

571 Cal per portion

Protein: 49g   Fat: 15.5g   Carbs: 52.1g

SERVES 2

Ingredients

2 rashers of smoked streaky bacon
120g dried pasta
Olive oil spray
1 tsp chopped garlic
1 white onion, diced
200g lean beef mince
1 tsp onion granules
½ tsp smoked paprika
1 tbsp Worcestershire sauce
½ tsp yellow American mustard
50g reduced-sugar ketchup
150ml hot beef stock
60g reduced-fat cheddar, grated
Salt and pepper
A few sprigs of fresh parsley, chopped, to garnish

Burger sauce drizzle

30g fat-free Greek yoghurt (you can sub this for lighter than light mayonnaise)
10g reduced-sugar ketchup
¼ tsp yellow American mustard
3 baby gherkins, diced
1 tsp gherkin juice

This is one of those recipes you can't help but come back to. Combining classic cheeseburger flavours with pasta, chopped bacon and a homemade burger sauce is a fusion of foods that tastes incredible. I use smoked streaky bacon here as that's what you usually get with a takeaway; however, you can use medallions or lean diced bacon bits instead to lower the calories.

Method

- Start by grilling the bacon according to the packet instructions. Once cooked, set to one side.

- Meanwhile, cook the pasta in a large pan of salted water according to the packet instructions. Once cooked, drain and set to one side.

- Spray a large frying pan with a few pumps of olive oil spray. Add the garlic and onion and cook for 2 minutes, then add the beef mince, frying over a high heat for 3-4 minutes until browned.

- Once the beef is brown, season with salt and pepper, the onion granules and smoked paprika before adding the Worcestershire sauce, mustard, ketchup and beef stock. Stir to combine, then bring to a simmer over a medium-high heat and leave for a few minutes until thickened.

- While the sauce thickens, mix together the burger sauce drizzle ingredients in a bowl.

- Once the sauce has thickened, stir through the cheese until melted. Remove the pan from the heat, add the cooked pasta and mix well.

- Cut the grilled bacon into small bits, then serve the pasta drizzled with the burger sauce, topped with the bacon bits and garnished with the parsley.

Speedy Cottage Pie Jacket Potato

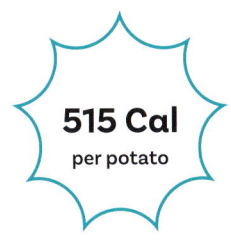

515 Cal per potato

Protein: 38.5g   **Fat: 11.1g**   **Carbs: 59.2g**

SERVES 2

Ingredients

2 large oblong-shaped baking potatoes (300g each)

Olive oil spray

1 small white onion, diced

1 tsp chopped garlic

200g lean beef mince

1 tbsp tomato purée

1 tbsp Worcestershire sauce

1 tsp mixed herb seasoning

1 beef stock cube, crumbled

150ml hot water

10g gravy granules

10g light butter

1 tbsp skimmed milk

20g reduced-fat cheddar, grated

Salt and pepper

2 sprigs of fresh parsley, chopped, to garnish

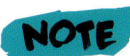

If you want a crispier potato, once you have topped it with the cheese, bake it in the oven for 15 minutes at 210°C/190°C fan or air fry it for 10 minutes at 190°C.

Who says you can't have a baked potato after a long day at work? I think we often overlook the mighty microwave and its powers. Granted, the skin isn't crispy compared to when you bake, but it will still bring you all the comfort.

Method

- Start by pricking the potatoes all over with a fork and spraying with a little olive oil spray before transferring to a microwavable plate.

- Season with salt and pepper and place in the microwave on high for 4 minutes (based on 1000W). After the 4 minutes is up, turn and cook for a further 4 minutes. Turn once more and cook for a final 2 minutes – the skin should look slightly shrivelled and the inside should feel very tender if pierced with a knife.

- Meanwhile, spray a large frying pan with olive oil spray. Over a high heat, fry the onion and garlic for a minute before adding the beef mince. Use a spatula to break up the mince.

- Once the mince is brown, add the tomato purée, Worcestershire sauce, herb seasoning, salt and pepper to taste, the crumbled stock cube and the water. Leave to reduce slightly for around a minute and a half before stirring through the gravy granules. Turn the heat down to low.

- Preheat the grill to high.

- Using an oven glove, carefully slice off the very top of each potato. Using a spoon, dig out the flesh and place it in a bowl. Season with a pinch of salt and pepper, add the butter and milk and mash with a fork. Don't worry if it isn't smooth, it needs texture to hold its shape.

- Scoop the beef mince inside the potato, pushing it down carefully. Top with the mash and push again slightly to pack it down before topping with the cheese. Place under a hot grill for 2 minutes so that the cheese melts.

- Serve with the parsley scattered over the top.

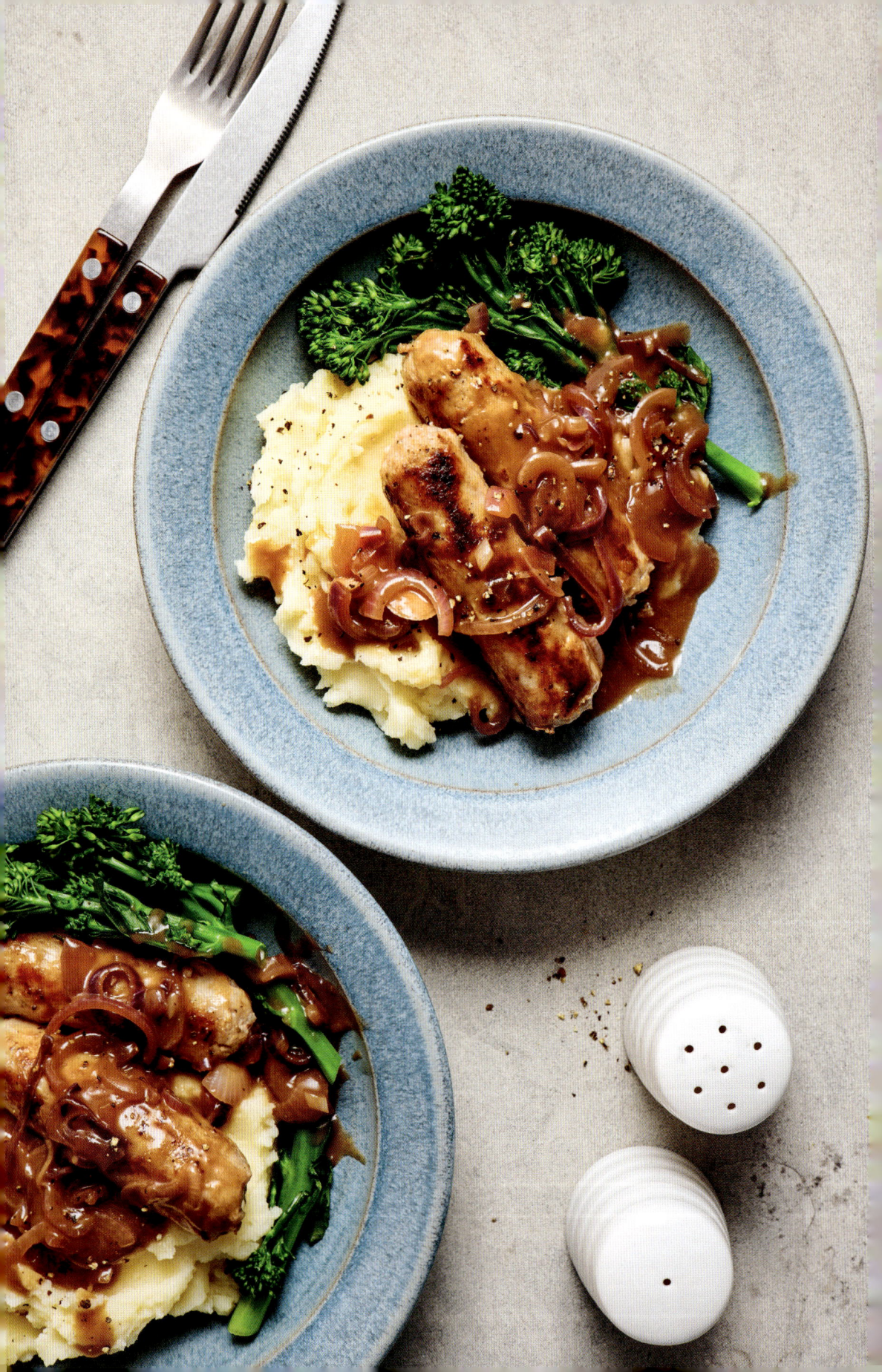

Bangers and Mash with Onion Gravy

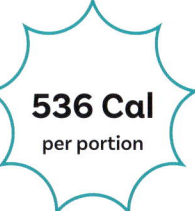

536 Cal per portion

Protein: 23.9g **Fat: 17.2g** **Carbs: 57.7g**

SERVES 2

Ingredients

4 reduced-fat pork sausages

500g Maris Piper potatoes, peeled and cubed

20g light butter, at room temperature

1 large red onion, sliced

½ tsp chopped garlic

15g plain flour

250ml beef stock

1 tsp onion granules

1 tbsp Worcestershire sauce

1 tbsp balsamic glaze

70ml semi-skimmed milk, gently warmed

Salt and pepper

For me there is no comfort food quite like this for dinner. Serve with a side of greens of your choice.

Method

- Preheat the grill to medium.
- Grill the sausages for around 16 minutes or according to your packet instructions, turning occasionally. You could also air fry them for 12–14 minutes at 185°C.
- Meanwhile, add the potatoes to a large pan of salted boiling water. Cook for 12–14 minutes until tender when pierced with a fork, then drain.
- While the above cook, heat a second saucepan over a medium-high heat. Melt 10g of the butter, then add the onion.
- Fry for a few minutes until the onion starts to soften, then add increments of 20ml water as needed to encourage the browning process.
- When the onion is soft and slightly brown, stir in the chopped garlic and cook for 30 seconds, then add the flour and stir until combined.
- Pour in the stock gradually, whisking constantly to combine.
- Once all of the stock is in the pan, season with salt and pepper, add the onion granules, Worcestershire sauce and balsamic glaze and leave to thicken over a medium heat until you have quite a thick, rich gravy.
- Season the drained potatoes well with salt and pepper, before adding the remaining butter and the milk. Use a potato masher to mash until smooth.
- Serve the mashed potato with the sausages on top. Pour the onion gravy all over.

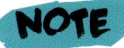

Store the sausages and gravy at one side of a container and the mash on the other side. Allow to cool before refrigerating. Reheat in the microwave on high for a few minutes until piping hot throughout. This will keep for a few days in the fridge. If you have an electric hand whisk, you can use this to make super-creamy potatoes.

Creamy Peppercorn Steak Potatoes

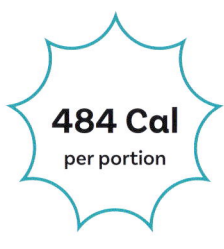

484 Cal per portion

| Protein: 32.7g | Fat: 14.3g | Carbs: 48.2g |

SERVES 2

AF

There is nothing quite like the combination of juicy bites of steak with a creamy peppercorn sauce, is there?

Ingredients

500g Maris Piper potatoes, peeled and cut into 2 x 1cm cubes

1 tsp dried parsley

1 tsp garlic granules

½ tsp dried rosemary

Olive oil spray

200g rump steak (or any of your choice)

1 tbsp Worcestershire sauce

1 white onion, diced

1½ tsp crushed peppercorns (if sensitive to spice, start with less and taste as you go)

1 tsp chopped garlic

100ml hot beef stock

100ml reduced-fat single cream alternative (I use Elmlea; or you can sub for reduced-fat crème fraîche)

15g Parmesan, grated

Salt and pepper

Method

- Start by patting the potato dry. Place in a large microwavable container and cook on full power for 3 minutes. Meanwhile, preheat the air fryer to 200°C.

- Once the time is up, transfer the potatoes straight to the air fryer basket. Season with the dried parsley, garlic granules and rosemary along with some salt and pepper. Spray generously with olive oil spray before giving it all a good shake. Air fry for 14 minutes until the potatoes are a light golden colour.

- Meanwhile, heat a large frying pan over a high heat. Season the steak on both sides with salt and pepper and place in the hot pan. Start by cooking for a minute on each side, then flipping for another 30 seconds on each side for medium-rare, or continue cooking until you have your desired level of cooked steak. Remove the steak from the pan and leave to rest.

- Meanwhile, deglaze the pan with the Worcestershire sauce, before adding the onion, crushed peppercorns and garlic. Fry for a couple of minutes before pouring in the beef stock and cream. Bring to a simmer and leave over a medium-high heat to reduce.

- While the sauce reduces, slice the steak into cubes.

- Remove the potatoes from the air fryer and divide equally between plates. Top with the cubes of steak along with the peppercorn sauce and the grated Parmesan.

Oven Place the potatoes onto a large baking tray in a preheated oven set at 220°C/200°C fan. Cook for 20-22 minutes, tossing partway through.

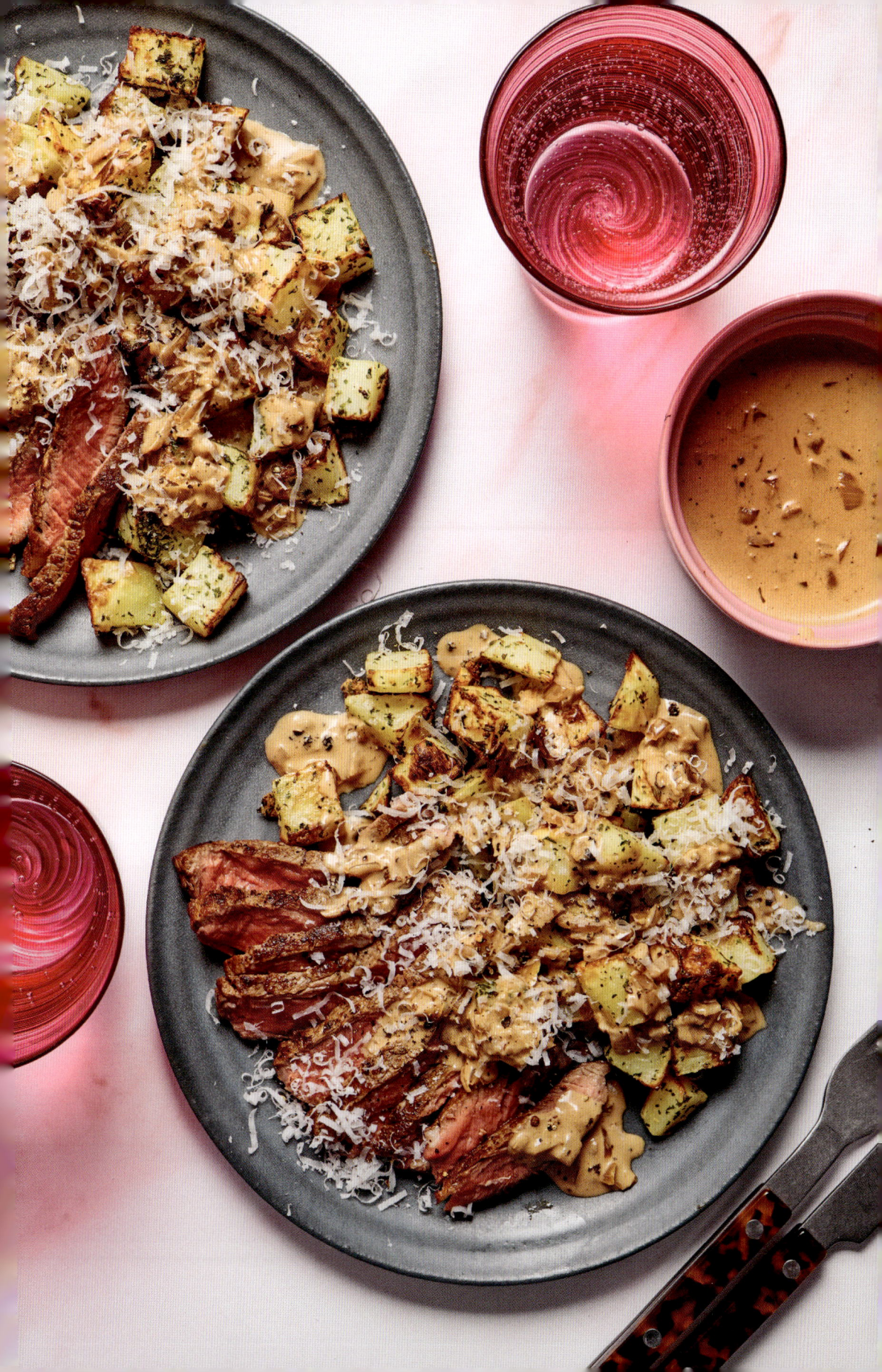

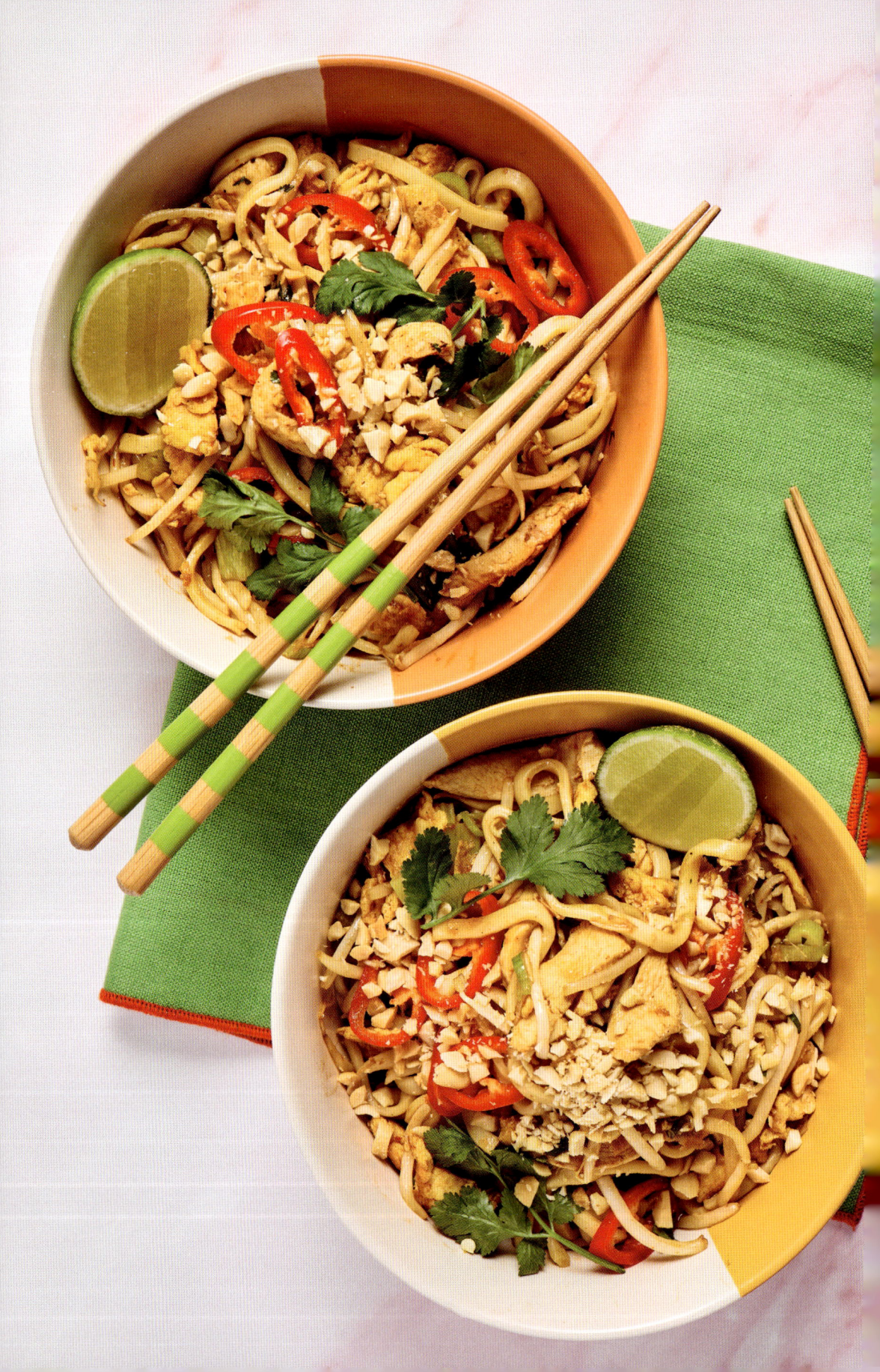

Pad Thai-Style Noodles

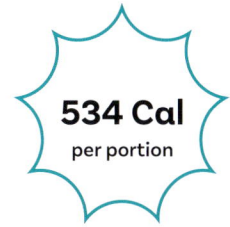

534 Cal per portion

| Protein: 46.5g | Fat: 13.1g | Carbs: 51.2g |

SERVES 2

How this dish takes me back to the busy Khao San Road with a backpack on my shoulders. Pad Thai is easily one of my favourite dishes from Thailand so it was only fitting to put my own version in this book. It's packed full of protein so it will help to keep those hunger cravings at bay. Swap the chicken for tofu for a veggie-friendly recipe.

Ingredients

Neutral cooking spray
200g skinless chicken breast, thinly sliced
2 medium eggs, whisked
1 heaped tsp chopped garlic
150g beansprouts
4 spring onions, chopped
2 × 150g packets of ready-to-wok wide noodles
2 sprigs of fresh coriander
15g peanuts, crushed
1 red chilli, sliced
2 slices of lime

Sauce
1½ tbsp tamarind paste
1 tbsp brown sugar
1½ tbsp fish sauce
1 tbsp oyster sauce
1 tbsp light soy sauce
1 tsp sriracha sauce
1 tsp lime juice
1 tbsp water

Method

- Start by heating a wok over a high heat. Spray with some cooking spray before adding the chicken. Fry for 6–7 minutes until cooked through, then remove from the pan.

- While the chicken cooks, mix together the ingredients for the sauce and set to one side.

- Turn down the heat under the wok slightly before pouring in the whisked eggs. Leave to set for 30 seconds before folding in and breaking up into pieces. Remove the egg from the pan and add it to the plate with the chicken.

- Spray the wok with a little more oil, then add the chopped garlic, beansprouts and half the spring onions and sauté for a couple of minutes.

- Add the noodles and cook for a couple more minutes.

- Move the noodles to one side before pouring in the sauce. Mix well to combine before adding the chicken and egg. Stir gently for a further minute to combine, then remove from the heat.

- Serve the noodles in bowls, topped with the remaining spring onions, the coriander, crushed peanuts, sliced chilli, if using, and a slice of lime for squeezing over.

Firecracker Salmon

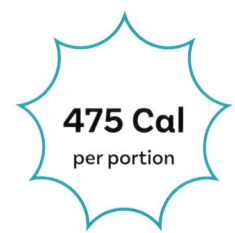

475 Cal per portion

Protein: 29.7g   **Fat: 13.2g**   **Carbs: 54.4g**

SERVES 2

This recipe is an explosion of flavour. A quick marinade is made with garlic, ginger, soy and sriracha sauce for the 'fire', along with brown sugar. This is then poured over salmon and baked for a flaky tender fillet. I find the heat of this fine, but if you struggle with spice, reduce the sriracha sauce by half, taste the sauce and increase if needed. If you are an anti-fish individual, this recipe is also banging with chicken! I like to serve this with Tenderstem broccoli or some pan-fried pak choi.

Ingredients

1 × 125g packet of boil-in-the-bag long-grain rice
1½ tsp chopped garlic
1 tsp ginger purée
30ml light soy sauce
20ml sriracha sauce
1 tsp brown sugar
½ tsp paprika
2 salmon fillets (260g in total), skin removed
½ tsp chilli flakes
2 spring onions, finely sliced

Sauce

40g lighter than light mayonnaise
15g reduced-sugar sweet chilli sauce
½ tsp sriracha sauce
1–2 tbsp hot water for desired consistency

Method

- Preheat the oven to 200°C/180°C fan.
- Cook the rice in a large pan of boiling water according to the packet instructions.
- In a bowl, mix together the garlic, ginger, soy sauce, sriracha sauce and brown sugar.
- Season the salmon fillets with the paprika and place into a baking dish. Pour the marinade all over the fillets and bake in the oven for 15 minutes.
- Meanwhile, make the sauce by combining the mayo, sweet chilli sauce and sriracha sauce. Use a tablespoon of hot water initially to loosen the mixture and create a thinner sauce. Use a further tablespoon if you prefer an even runnier sauce.
- Once the salmon is cooked, remove from the oven. Serve the salmon over the cooked rice, drizzled with the sauce and sprinkled with the chilli flakes and spring onions.

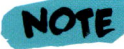

To remove the salmon skin more quickly, place the fillets skin-side up on a wire rack and run under hot water. After a minute, the ends of the skin should shrivel slightly and you can peel the skin off. Pat dry with kitchen paper.

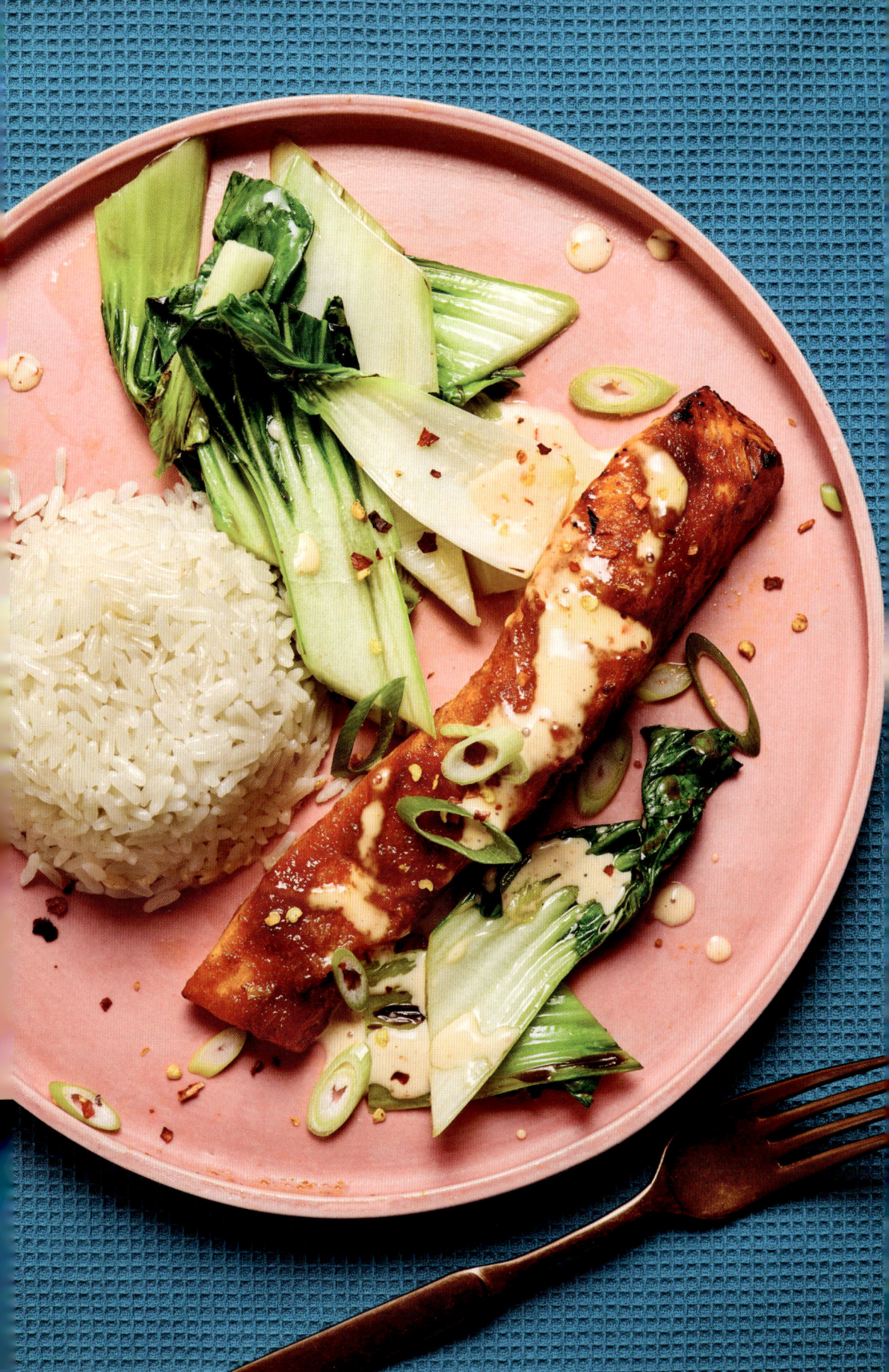

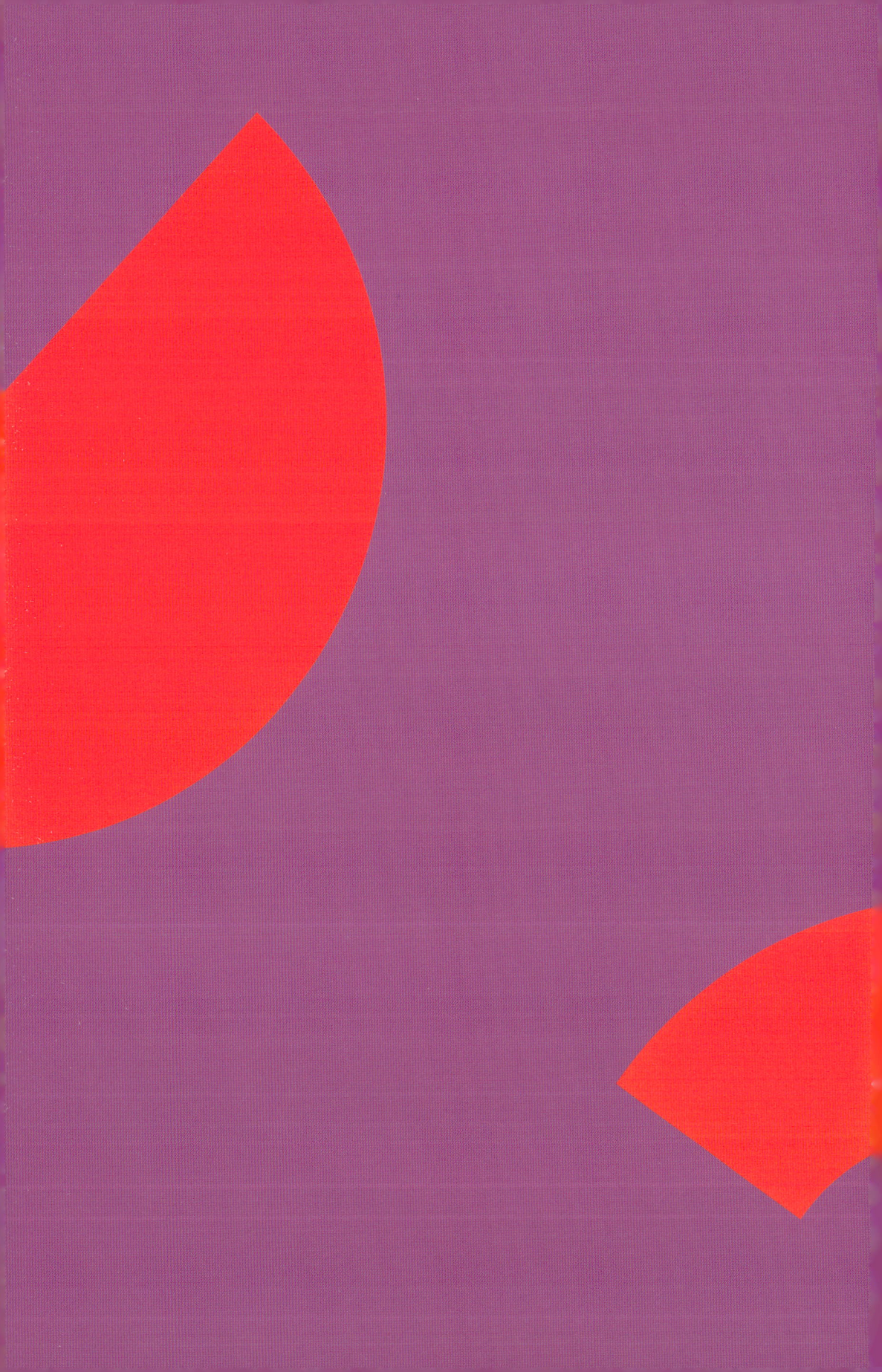

Six

SPEEDY FAKEAWAYS

Salmon Yakitori

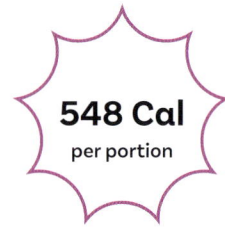

548 Cal per portion

Protein: 30.3g Fat: 13.2g Carbs: 72.1g

SERVES 2

Ingredients

1 × 125g packet of boil-in-the-bag long-grain rice

2 × salmon fillets, (260g in total), skin removed and cut into 2.5cm cubes

1 tsp smoked paprika

1 tsp garlic granules

50ml light soy sauce

20g brown sugar

30ml mirin

1 tsp chopped ginger

1 tsp chopped garlic

4 spring onions, cut into 5cm strips

½ tsp white sesame seeds

½ tsp black sesame seeds

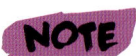

You can also fry the skewers. Spray a large frying pan with a few pumps of neutral cooking spray and cook over a medium-high heat for 6 minutes, carefully turning them partway through, until cooked through.

This is one of my favourite foods from when I backpacked in Japan. The sauce is made up of soy sauce, brown sugar and mirin, and I also like to add some ginger and garlic for an irresistible flavour. Traditionally this is made with chicken so feel free to make it with chicken, though it is just as banging with salmon. You could also throw it on top of some noodles rather than rice.

Method

- Cook the rice in a large pan of boiling water according to the packet instructions.
- Preheat the grill to high.
- Put the salmon into a bowl and season with the smoked paprika and garlic granules.
- To a separate bowl, add the soy sauce, brown sugar, mirin, ginger and garlic and whisk to combine. Pour a quarter over the salmon and mix well.
- Thread the salmon and spring onion strips onto small metal skewers. If you have wooden ones, soak them for 30 minutes prior to cooking to prevent them from burning.
- Place the skewers on a grill tray under the hot grill, pouring over any leftover sauce that was in the bowl with the salmon. Cook for 6 minute, turning partway through.
- Meanwhile, put the remaining sauce into a saucepan and leave to simmer over a low heat to thicken.
- Once the rice has cooked, carefully cut the bag and divide between two bowls. Top with the salmon skewers and the thickened sauce from the pan.
- Garnish with the white and black sesame seeds.

Air Fryer Place the skewers in the air fryer and cook for 6–8 minutes at 180°C.

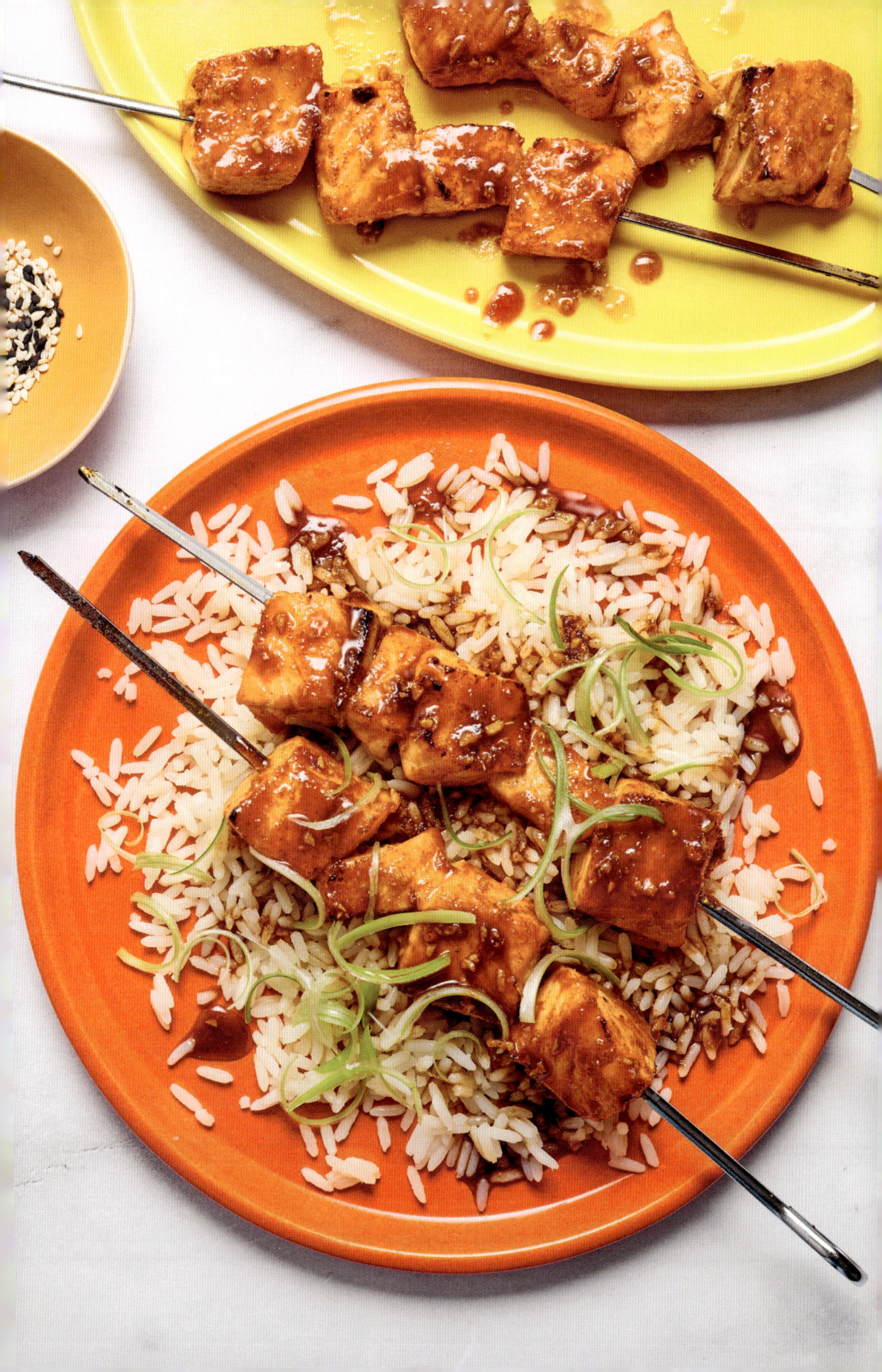

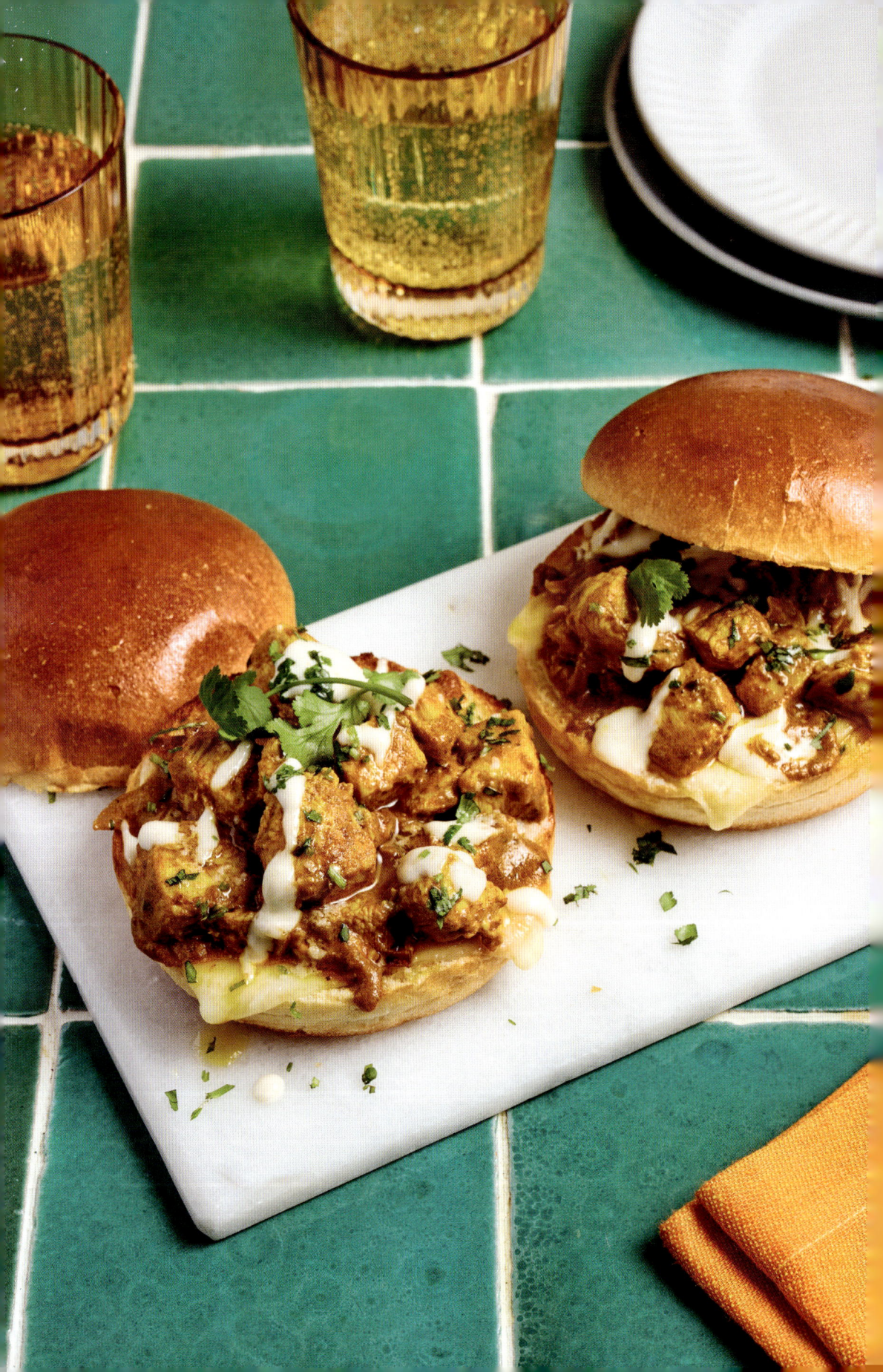

Chicken Tikka Buns

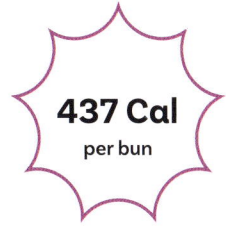

437 Cal per bun

Protein: 41.2g **Fat: 13.8g** **Carbs: 34.1g**

MAKES 4

These tikka buns are a fun way to spice up that weekend dinner. Chicken tikka is loaded into a garlic-butter-brushed bun with melted cheese and garlic mayo. With all dishes like this, if you have the opportunity to marinate the chicken prior to cooking, please do. If not, don't worry, it will still taste banging!

Ingredients

400g skinless chicken breast, cut into small cubes
1 tbsp garam masala
50g tikka paste
40g fat-free natural yoghurt
1 tbsp lemon juice
Olive oil spray
2 tsp chopped garlic
1 tsp ginger purée
1 red onion, diced
4 brioche buns
4 mozzarella slices
A few sprigs of fresh coriander, chopped
10g light butter

Garlic mayo
50g lighter than light mayonnaise
1 tsp garlic granules
1 tsp lemon juice
Pinch of salt

Method

- Start by preheating the oven to 210°C/190°C fan.
- Next, add the chicken to a bowl and season with the garam masala. Add the tikka paste, along with the yoghurt and lemon juice. Stir to combine.
- Spray a large frying pan with a few pumps of olive oil spray. Over a medium–high heat, add 1 teaspoon of the chopped garlic and the ginger, followed by the chicken. Fry for 8–9 minutes, until cooked through, then add the onion for a couple more minutes to soften.
- While the chicken cooks, mix together the ingredients for the garlic mayo and set to one side. Then, toast the bottom buns of the brioche in a toaster until slightly golden.
- Place the bottom buns on a baking tray. Top with the mozzarella slices, followed by the chicken, garlic mayo and coriander, then finish with the tops of the buns. Bake for 4–5 minutes, until the cheese has melted.
- Put the remaining teaspoon of chopped garlic into a microwavable bowl along with the butter and blast in the microwave on medium for 15–20 seconds until melted, stirring to combine.
- Once the cheese has melted, remove the buns from the oven and brush the garlic butter over the tops to serve.

Vegetable Gyoza Noodle Bowls

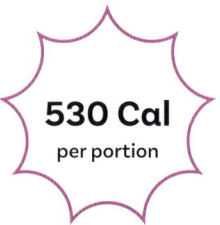

530 Cal per portion

| Protein: 16.1g | Fat: 22.7g | Carbs: 57.8g |

SERVES 2

Fragrant, zesty and hearty, these noodle bowls are banging. I don't know about you but there is something so comforting about slurping up a tasty broth. Here the flavours are Thai-inspired, with red curry paste as the base of the sauce. The base of this recipe is also delicious with shredded chicken added too, for a protein hit, or even a jammy egg.

Ingredients

50g red curry paste
1 tsp chopped garlic
1 tsp chopped ginger
400ml light coconut milk
500ml hot vegetable stock (made with 2 cubes)
1 tbsp light soy sauce
1 tbsp lime juice
Neutral cooking spray
8 frozen vegetable gyoza dumplings
1 pak choi, chopped
2 × 150g packets of ready-to-wok medium noodles
1 tsp chilli oil (optional)
2 sprigs of fresh coriander, chopped
½ tsp black sesame seeds

Method

- Put the red curry paste, garlic and ginger into a saucepan over a medium heat and leave for a minute.

- Pour in the coconut milk, 400ml of the vegetable stock, the soy sauce and lime juice. Cook over a high heat for 10 minutes.

- Meanwhile, spray a large frying pan (that has a lid) with cooking spray. Add the gyozas and fry over a medium heat for 3 minutes or until the bottoms are crispy. Pour in the remaining stock and cover for around 5 minutes, until the liquid has dissolved, then remove from the heat.

- Once the 10 minutes of cooking time on the broth is up, add the pak choi and noodles and simmer for half their recommended time, stirring here and there until they loosen.

- Pour the liquid into deep bowls, then add the noodles followed by the crispy gyoza.

- Garnish with the chilli oil, if using, the chopped coriander and the sesame seeds.

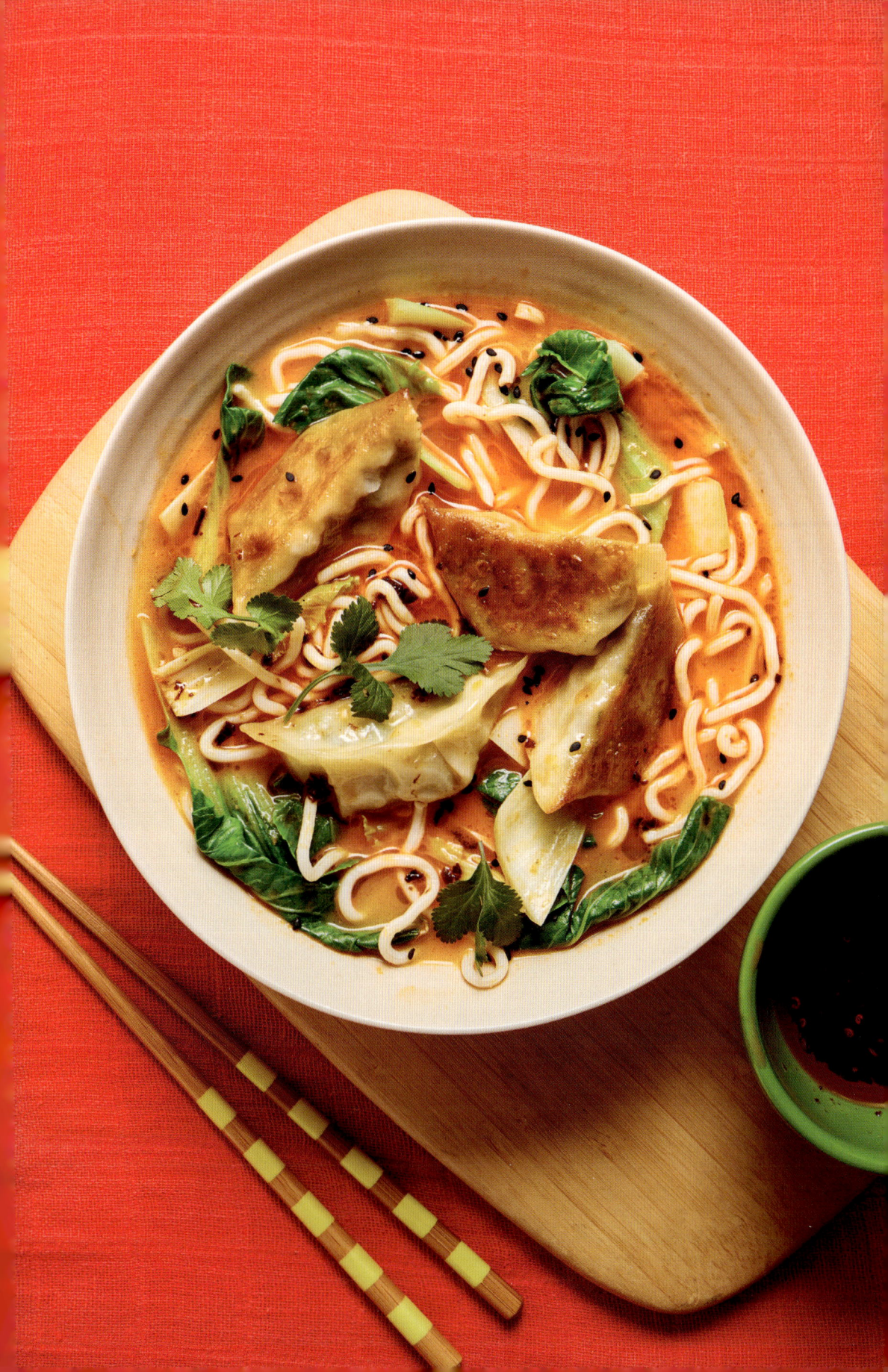

Bang Bang Chicken Banh Mi

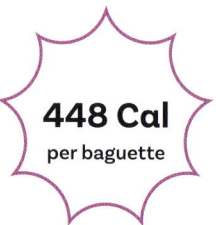

448 Cal per baguette

Protein: 38.1g   **Fat: 4.8g**   **Carbs: 60.5g**

SERVES 2

If you've ever visited Vietnam, I'm sure you've been in the banh mi chokehold. This recipe isn't authentic, but I have borrowed some of the gorgeous parts from the traditional sandwich and have given it a kitchen bangers twist. Trust me, you will love this version.

Ingredients

200g skinless chicken breast, thinly sliced

1 tsp chopped garlic

1 tsp chopped ginger

1 tsp paprika

1 tbsp light soy sauce

1 tsp fish sauce

2 × 100g bake-at-home crusty white baguettes

Neutral cooking spray

40g lighter than light mayonnaise

15g sweet chilli sauce

1 tsp sriracha sauce

1 small carrot, grated

3 sprigs of fresh coriander, roughly chopped

Quick pickled vegetables

2 tbsp rice wine vinegar

¼ tsp white sugar

¼ tsp sea salt

2 radishes, sliced

½ small red onion, sliced

100ml warm water

Method

- Start by putting the sliced chicken into a bowl. Add the garlic, ginger, paprika, soy sauce and fish sauce. Give it all a good stir to combine.

- Put all of the ingredients for the pickled vegetables into a jar and set to one side.

- Bake the baguettes as per the packet instructions.

- Heat a large frying pan over a medium-high heat. Spray with a few pumps of cooking spray.

- Once hot, add the sliced chicken. Cook for 8 minutes or until cooked through.

- Meanwhile, to a small bowl, add the mayo, sweet chilli sauce and sriracha sauce to make the bang bang sauce. Mix to combine. If the sauce is really thick, add a teaspoon of hot water to loosen it slightly.

- Once the baguettes are cooked, slice them open. Spread half of the bang bang sauce on the bottom and then top with the cooked chicken slices.

- Top with the pickled vegetables, grated carrot, the remaining bang bang sauce and the coriander.

Garlic Aioli Steak Sandwiches

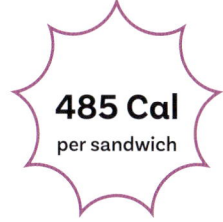
485 Cal per sandwich

Protein: 37g **Fat: 18.4g** **Carbs: 42.8g**

SERVES 2

Switch up that steak night with these banging sandwiches. Juicy steak is layered onto a light ciabatta roll with a homemade garlic aioli sauce, rocket and cheese. You can serve these with a crunchy balsamic salad with juicy tomatoes, or make some homemade chips to go with them.

Ingredients

10g light butter
1 white onion, sliced
200g rump steak (or any of your choice)
Olive oil spray
2 bake-at-home ciabatta rolls
2 reduced-fat cheddar slices
2 handfuls of rocket
10ml balsamic glaze (optional)
Salt and pepper

Garlic aioli sauce
45g fat-free Greek yoghurt
20g lighter than light mayonnaise
1 tsp lemon juice
½ tsp garlic granules
¼ tsp chopped garlic

Method

- Preheat the oven according to the packet instructions for the ciabatta rolls.
- Start by melting the butter in a saucepan. Once melted, add the onion and cook over a low heat.
- Meanwhile, season the steak all over with salt and pepper.
- Spray a large frying pan with a few pumps of olive oil spray. Leave to heat over a high heat, then add the steak. Cook for a minute each side, then a further 30 seconds on each side for medium-rare. Cook the steak for a further 2 minutes or so if you like yours more cooked.
- Remove from the pan and set to one side to rest.
- Place the ciabatta rolls in the oven and bake according to the packet instructions.
- Check on the onions and add a splash of water (in increments) to help them to brown, giving them a good stir.
- While the onions brown, make the garlic aioli sauce by mixing together all the ingredients, then set to one side.
- Slice the ciabatta rolls in half, place the cheese slices on the top halves and put all the pieces back in the oven for a minute for the cheese to melt and the bare sides to toast a little.
- Meanwhile, slice the steak thinly. In a bowl, toss the rocket with the balsamic glaze, if using.
- Add half the garlic aioli to the bottom of the ciabattas, topping with the rocket, steak, cooked onions and the remaining garlic aioli, then cover with the cheesy ciabatta halves.

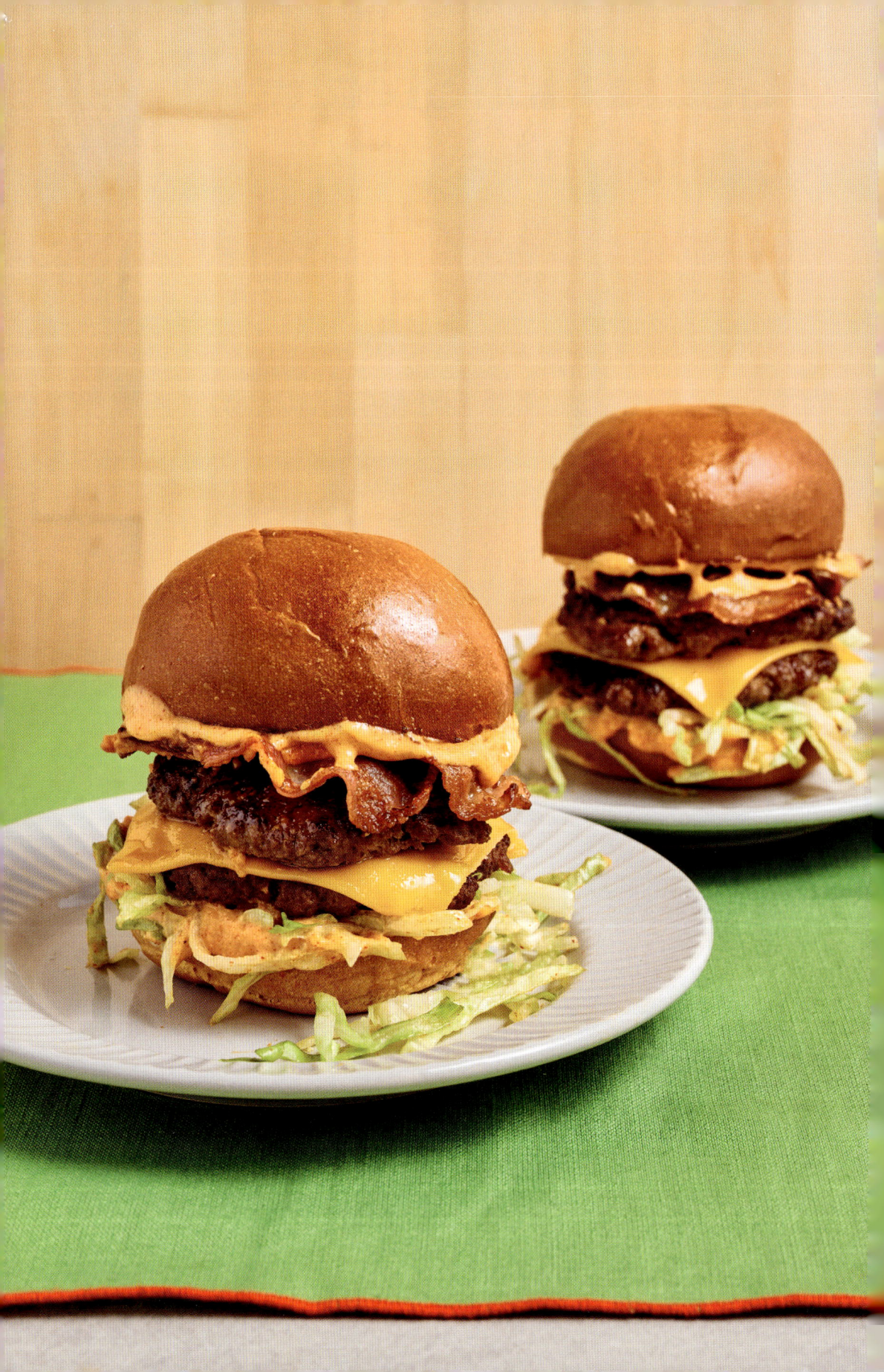

Baconnaise Double Cheeseburgers

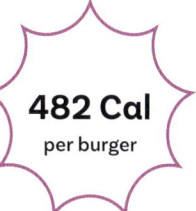

482 Cal per burger

Protein: 47.2g **Fat: 17.7g** **Carbs: 30.5g**

SERVES 2

Your next banging burger recipe is here and it's full of smoky bacon flavours. Two burger patties are smashed down and topped with cheese, then piled onto a toasted brioche bun with a tasty homemade baconnaise sauce and extra bacon for good measure. I really recommend sticking to streaky bacon for the best flavour, but you can use bacon medallions if you wish.

Ingredients

4 rashers of smoked streaky bacon
250g 5% lean beef mince
1 tsp garlic granules
1 tsp onion granules
35g lighter than light mayonnaise
5g reduced-sugar ketchup
¼ tsp smoked paprika
¼ tsp yellow American mustard
1 tsp distilled white vinegar
Olive oil spray
2 light cheese slices
2 brioche buns
2 handfuls of shredded lettuce
1 tsp bacon bits (optional)
Salt and pepper

Method

- Start by grilling the bacon according to the packet instructions over a grill tray lined with foil.

- Meanwhile, season the beef with the garlic granules, onion granules and some salt and pepper. Combine everything well before splitting the mince into four equal balls. Leave to one side.

- Next, put the mayo, ketchup, smoked paprika, mustard, distilled white vinegar and 1 teaspoon of water into a bowl. Mix until well combined, then set to one side until the bacon has cooked.

- Heat frying pan sprayed with a few pumps of olive oil spray over a medium-high heat. Add the beef balls and, using a spatula or burger press, flatten down each ball into a patty. Fry for 2 minutes each side or until browned and cooked through, then turn the heat down to low, add the cheese slices to two of the patties, top with the remaining patties and leave the cheese to melt.

- Meanwhile, toast the brioche buns until lightly golden.

- At this point, the bacon should be cooked. Chop two rashers of bacon into small pieces. Stir through the mayo sauce made earlier and pour the bacon fat into the sauce.

- Spread half the mayo sauce over the bottom of each bun. Top with the shredded lettuce, followed by the burger patties, the remaining sauce, the cooked bacon rashers, and the crispy bacon bits if using.

Nacho Beef Folded Wraps

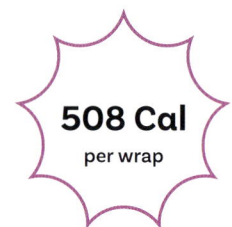

508 Cal per wrap

Protein: 38.7g   Fat: 17.1g   Carbs: 43.8g

SERVES 2

If you follow me on social media, you know that I love a folded wrap. This combination is one of my all-time favourites and I am sure it will be one of yours too. Taco beef is folded with shredded lettuce, nacho cheese dip and tortilla chips for an absolute whopper of a wrap. Serve with a side salad or, if you're extra hungry, some Mexican flavoured rice.

Ingredients

Olive oil spray
1 red onion diced
1 tsp chopped garlic
200g lean beef mince
1 tbsp taco seasoning
1 tbsp tomato salsa
50ml water
2 tortilla wraps
2 handfuls of shredded lettuce
15g tortilla chips (I use Chilli Heatwave Doritos)
40g nacho cheese dip
30g reduced-fat cheddar, grated

Method

- Start by spraying a medium frying pan with olive oil spray. Fry the onion and garlic for a minute over a high heat, then add the mince and fry for around 5 minutes, until browned, adding the taco seasoning once it has almost browned. Mix well to combine, before adding the salsa and water. Turn the heat down slightly.
- Heat a large clean frying pan with no oil over a medium heat.
- Next, microwave the wraps on high for 15 seconds before slicing partway down the middle.
- Pile the lettuce into one quarter of each wrap, then the taco beef into another quarter, ensuring it is squashed down, then the tortilla chips in a third quarter. Spread 15g of nacho cheese dip on the final quarter and top it with the grated cheese, then dollop the remaining nacho cheese dip on top of the beef.
- Carefully fold each section over itself, finishing with the cheese section.
- Add the wraps to the clean pan, placing them cheese-side down, and heat for around 1½ minutes before flipping for a further minute or until slightly crispy.

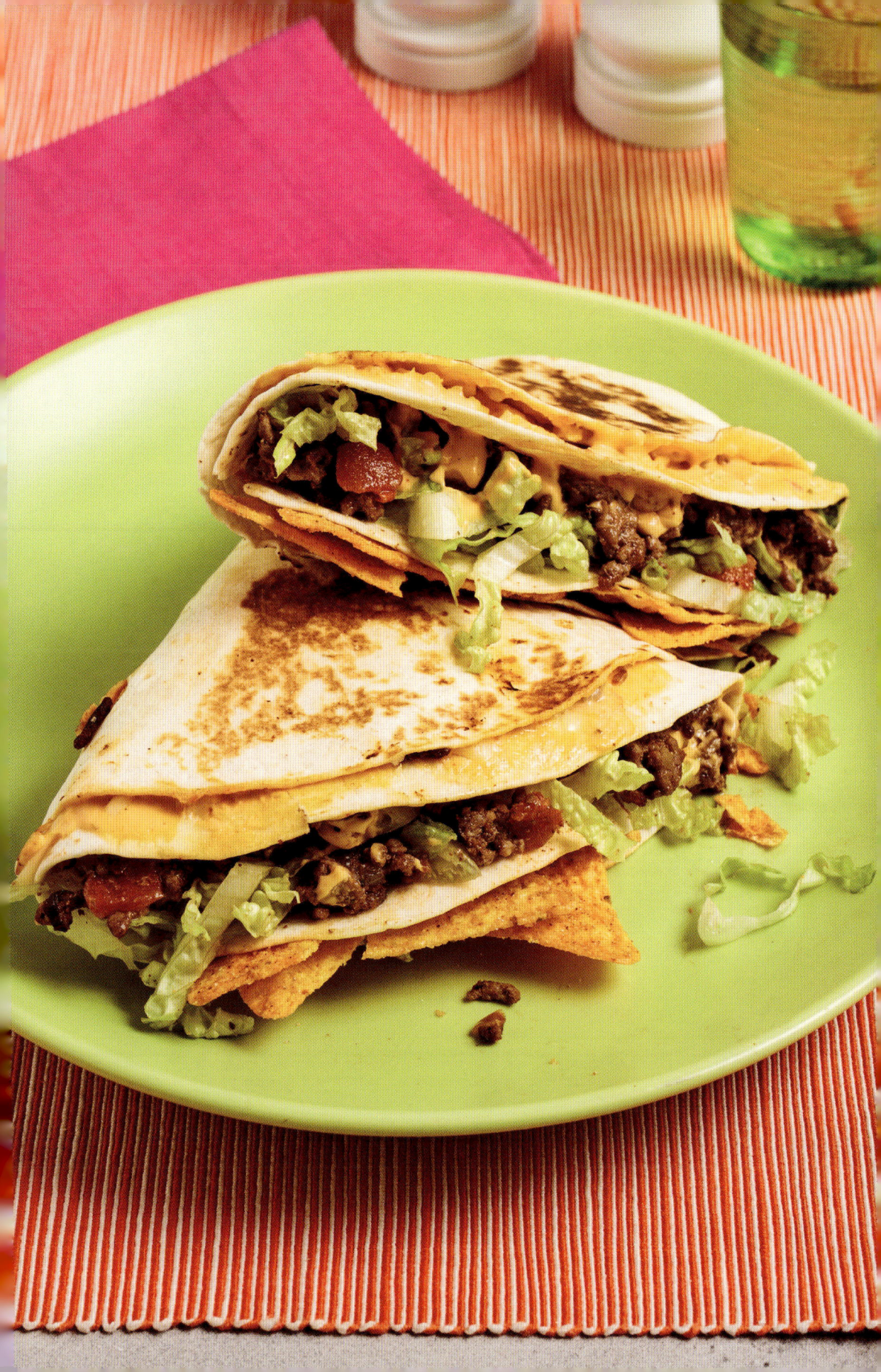

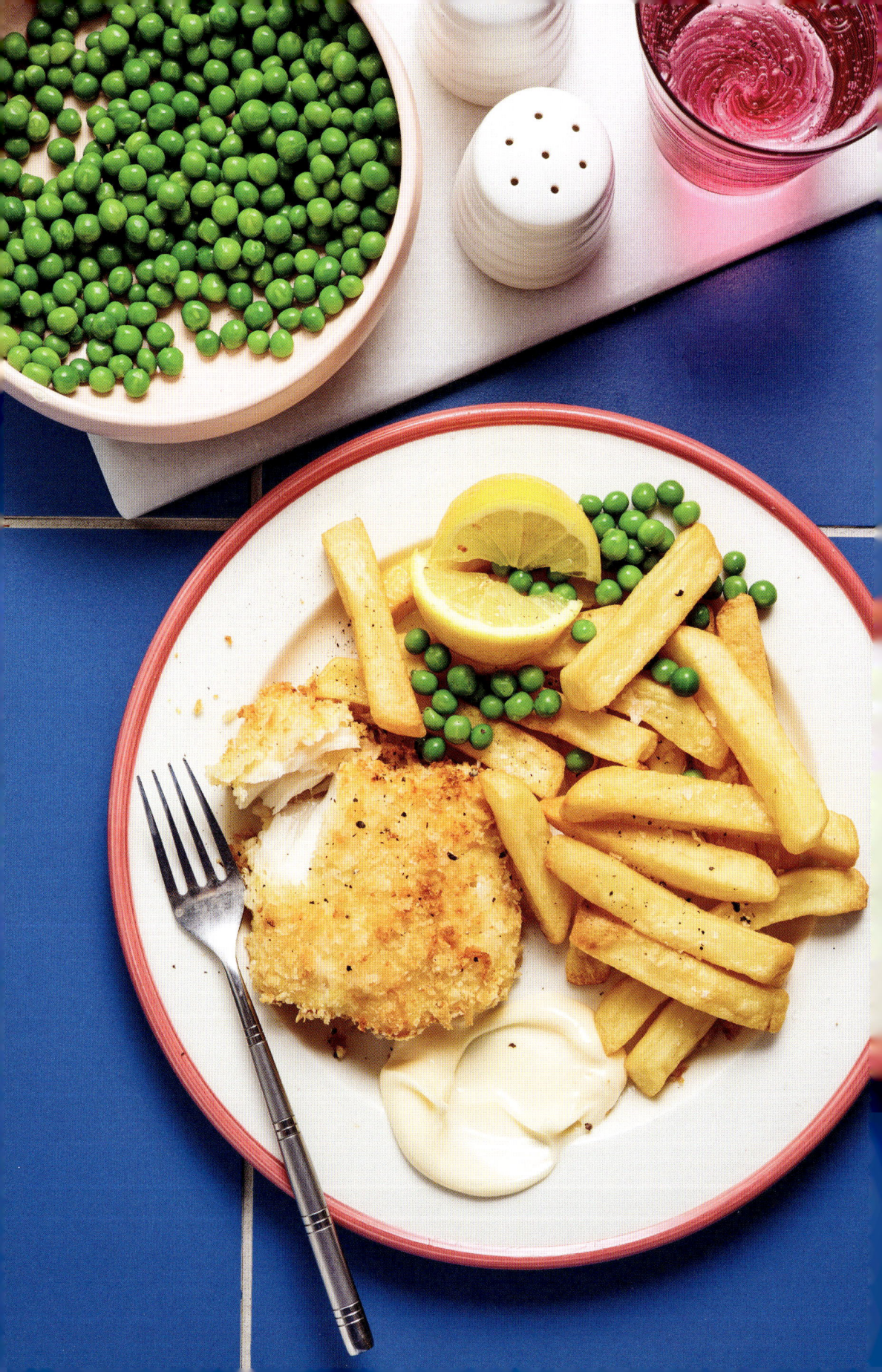

Lemon Pepper Parmesan Fish and Chips

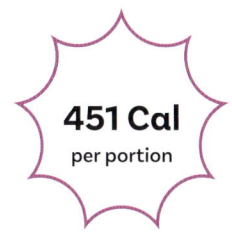

451 Cal per portion

Protein: 32.8g **Fat: 7g** **Carbs: 60.5g**

SERVES 2

This book had to have fish and chips but I wanted to jazz it up a little. I may be biased but this is the best home-cooked fish I have ever had. The breadcrumbs are seasoned with lemon zest, grated Parmesan and cracked black pepper for the most delicious golden crunchy coating. It's served alongside chips and a tasty lemon garlic sauce (add some peas if you wish) for a fancy dinner at home. Feel free to use any white fish you like.

Ingredients

2 × 140g skinless cod loin fillets
1½ tsp garlic granules
1 tsp onion granules
40g panko breadcrumbs
Zest and juice of 1 lemon
10g Parmesan, grated
1 medium egg, whisked
300g frozen lighter home chips
40g lighter than light mayonnaise
Salt and cracked black pepper

Method

- Start by preheating the air fryer to 200°C.
- Pat the cod fillets dry on both sides with kitchen paper. Season on both sides with 1 teaspoon of the garlic granules, the onion granules and some salt and pepper.
- Season the breadcrumbs with the lemon zest, Parmesan and ¼ teaspoon of cracked black pepper and toss to combine.
- Dip each cod fillet into the egg, ensuring it is all coated. Shake off any excess before dipping into the breadcrumbs. Push the breadcrumbs gently into the fish to adhere.
- Place the fish directly in the air fryer basket, along with the chips, for 14 minutes, turning partway through.
- While the fish cooks, make the sauce by combining the mayo, remaining ½ teaspoon of garlic granules, the lemon juice and salt and pepper to taste. Pour into two sauce dishes.
- Once the fish is cooked, squeeze over any remaining lemon juice and serve on plates with the chips and sauce.

Oven Place the fish fillets onto a baking tray and bake in the centre of a preheated oven set to 220°C/200°C fan for 18–20 minutes.

Lamb Shish Kebabs

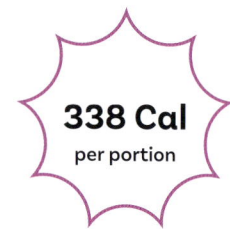

338 Cal per portion

| Protein: 38.6g | Fat: 15.4g | Carbs: 7.3g |

SERVES 2

These Turkish-inspired lamb kebabs will help you to ditch those takeaways and keep you on track with your weight loss goals. If you do have time to marinate this lamb, I will always recommend doing so, to enhance the flavours. Serve either with a big salad, drizzled with garlic and herb sauce, or pop it all inside a soft pitta bread with some chilli sauce.

Ingredients

250g boneless lamb leg steaks, at room temperature, cut into chunks

½ tsp smoked paprika

½ tsp ground cumin

½ tsp dried oregano

½ tsp sumac

1 tsp chopped garlic

1 white onion, grated

1 tsp tomato purée

1 tbsp lemon juice

1 tbsp fat-free natural yoghurt

1 red pepper, cut into chunks

1 green pepper, cut into chunks

1 red onion, cut into chunks

Olive oil spray

Salt and pepper

Method

- Preheat the oven to 220ºC/200ºC fan.
- Put the lamb into a bowl and season with the smoked paprika, cumin, oregano, sumac and some salt and pepper. Then add the garlic, grated onion, tomato purée, lemon juice and yoghurt and mix all of the ingredients together.
- To assemble the skewers, use metal skewers preferably. If you use wooden skewers, soak them for 30 minutes prior to cooking to prevent them from burning. Thread the peppers, red onion and lamb chunks onto the skewers. Place on a baking tray sprayed with olive oil spray and bake in the oven for 12 minutes.
- Once cooked, remove from the oven and serve.

Air fryer Preheat the air fryer to 200ºC and spray the basket with olive oil spray. Place the skewers inside and cook for 8–10 minutes, turning partway through.

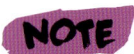

You can leave the sumac out if you wish, though it does add a nice zest to the recipe!

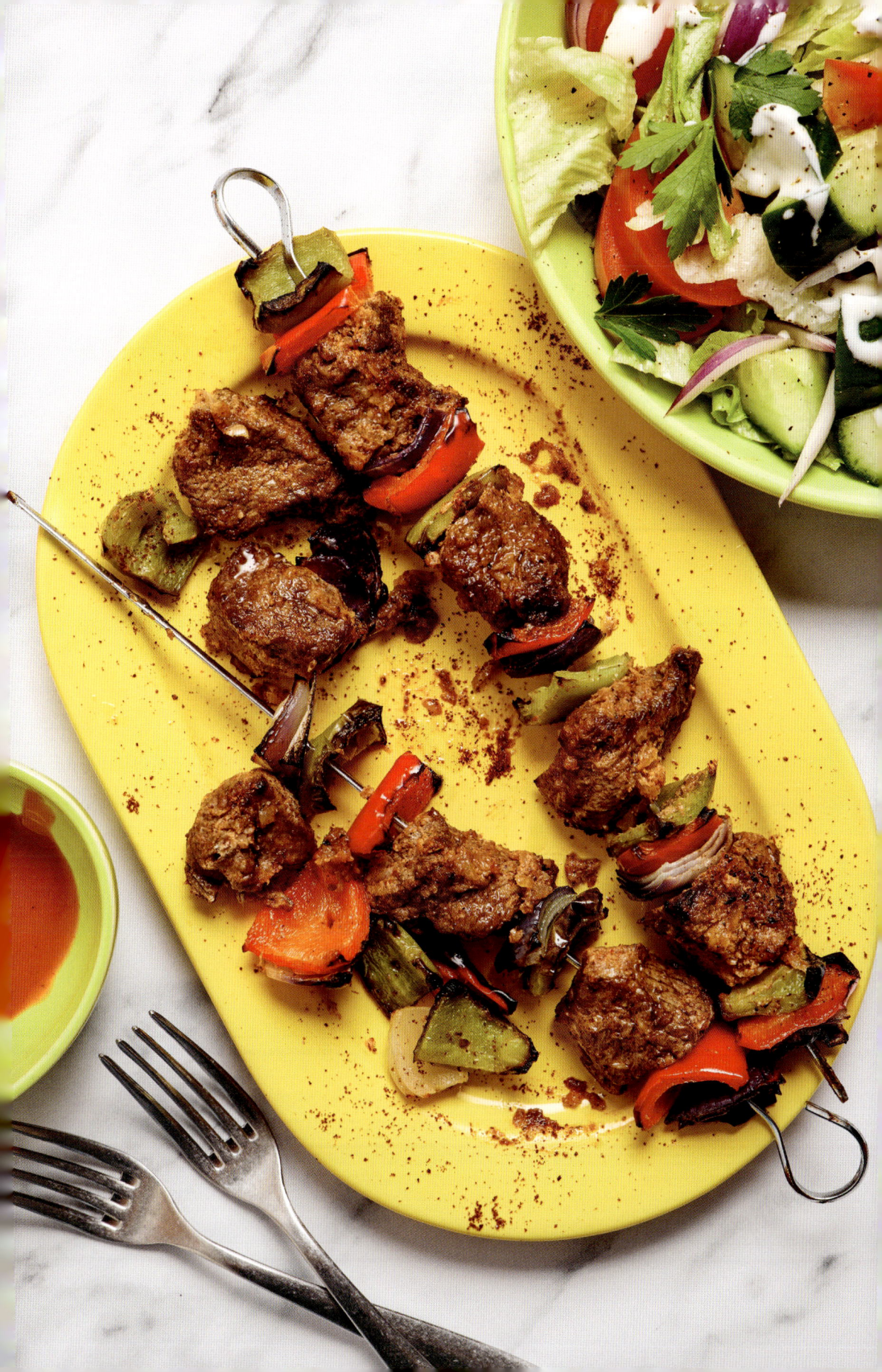

BBQ Shredded Chicken Cajun Fries

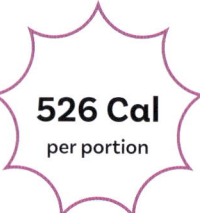

526 Cal per portion

| Protein: 38.3g | Fat: 12.9g | Carbs: 60g |

SERVES 2

 AF

When those busy nights come calling, let the oven do the work for you. This is a really easy yet banging dinner made up of Cajun-seasoned frozen fries, along with shredded barbecue chicken, a quick nacho cheese sauce and extra Cajun seasoning to dust. This is heavenly with a crisp balsamic-glazed salad, and if you have the calories to spare, I urge you to drizzle some ranch sauce over the fries, too.

Ingredients

350g crispy skin-on frozen fries

1 tsp Cajun seasoning, plus extra to finish

200g skinless chicken breast, cut into strips

1½ tsp barbecue seasoning

1 tsp smoked paprika

40g barbecue sauce

2 light cheese slices

3 tbsp semi-skimmed milk

Method

- Preheat the oven to 240°C/220°C fan.
- Put the fries onto a large baking tray. Season with the Cajun seasoning and toss to ensure all the fries are coated. Place in the oven and cook according to the packet instructions (mine take around 17 minutes).
- Next, place the chicken strips on a separate baking tray. Season with the barbecue seasoning and smoked paprika and rub them in thoroughly before placing in the oven for 12 minutes, until cooked through.
- Once the chicken has cooked, remove from the oven. Transfer to a chopping board and shred using two forks. Squeeze over the barbecue sauce and mix with the chicken.
- Place the cheese slices and milk in a microwavable bowl and leave to one side.
- Once the fries are cooked, remove from the oven. Blast the cheese in the microwave on high for 15-20 seconds, stirring with a fork to combine.
- Serve the shredded chicken on top of the fries and pour the sauce all over. Finish with a dusting of Cajun seasoning.

Air Fryer To cook the fries, check the packet instructions, but they usually take around 10-12 minutes at 190°C. Cook the chicken at 220°C for 8-10 minutes or until cooked through.

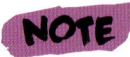

Make sure you use fries that can be cooked quickly – some take longer than others.

Chicken Shawarma Flatbreads

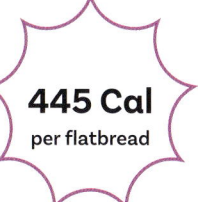
445 Cal per flatbread

| Protein: 38.6g | Fat: 5g | Carbs: 60.4g |

SERVES 2

This recipe is guaranteed to shock your tastebuds. There is so much flavour packed in every single bite, from the charred pan-fried chicken, to the crisp and tangy sumac onions, garlic yoghurt sauce and fresh salad.

Ingredients

200g skinless chicken breast, cut into thin slices
½ tsp ground cumin
½ tsp paprika
½ tsp ground turmeric
¼ tsp ground cinnamon
½ tsp garlic powder
1 tbsp tomato purée
1 tbsp lemon juice
Olive oil spray
2 Lebanese flatbreads (I use white Dina Paninette)
1 × 130g bag of shredded lettuce
2 salad tomatoes, sliced
1 tbsp sriracha sauce
Salt and pepper

Sumac onions
1 red onion
¾ tsp sumac
1 tbsp lemon juice
2 sprigs of fresh parsley, chopped
Pinch of salt

Garlic sauce
60g fat-free Greek yoghurt
½ tsp chopped garlic
½ tsp lemon juice
Pinch of salt

Method

- Start by putting the sliced chicken into a bowl. Season with salt and pepper to taste, the cumin, paprika, turmeric, cinnamon and garlic powder, before adding the tomato purée and lemon juice. Give everything a good stir and set to one side.
- Spray a large frying pan with olive oil spray and set over a medium-high heat.
- While the pan heats, put add all of the ingredients for the sumac onions into a separate bowl and leave to one side.
- Add the chicken to the frying pan, ensuring each piece is separated. Leave undisturbed for 2 minutes before flipping and repeating. This will help to get a nice char effect on the chicken. Continue to cook for 6 minutes, flipping occasionally, until cooked through.
- Meanwhile, make the garlic sauce by mixing together all the ingredients.
- Once the chicken has cooked, grab the flatbreads and top with the garlic sauce, spreading it out to cover the surface. Top with the lettuce, tomatoes, cooked chicken and sumac onions. Finish by drizzling over the sriracha sauce.

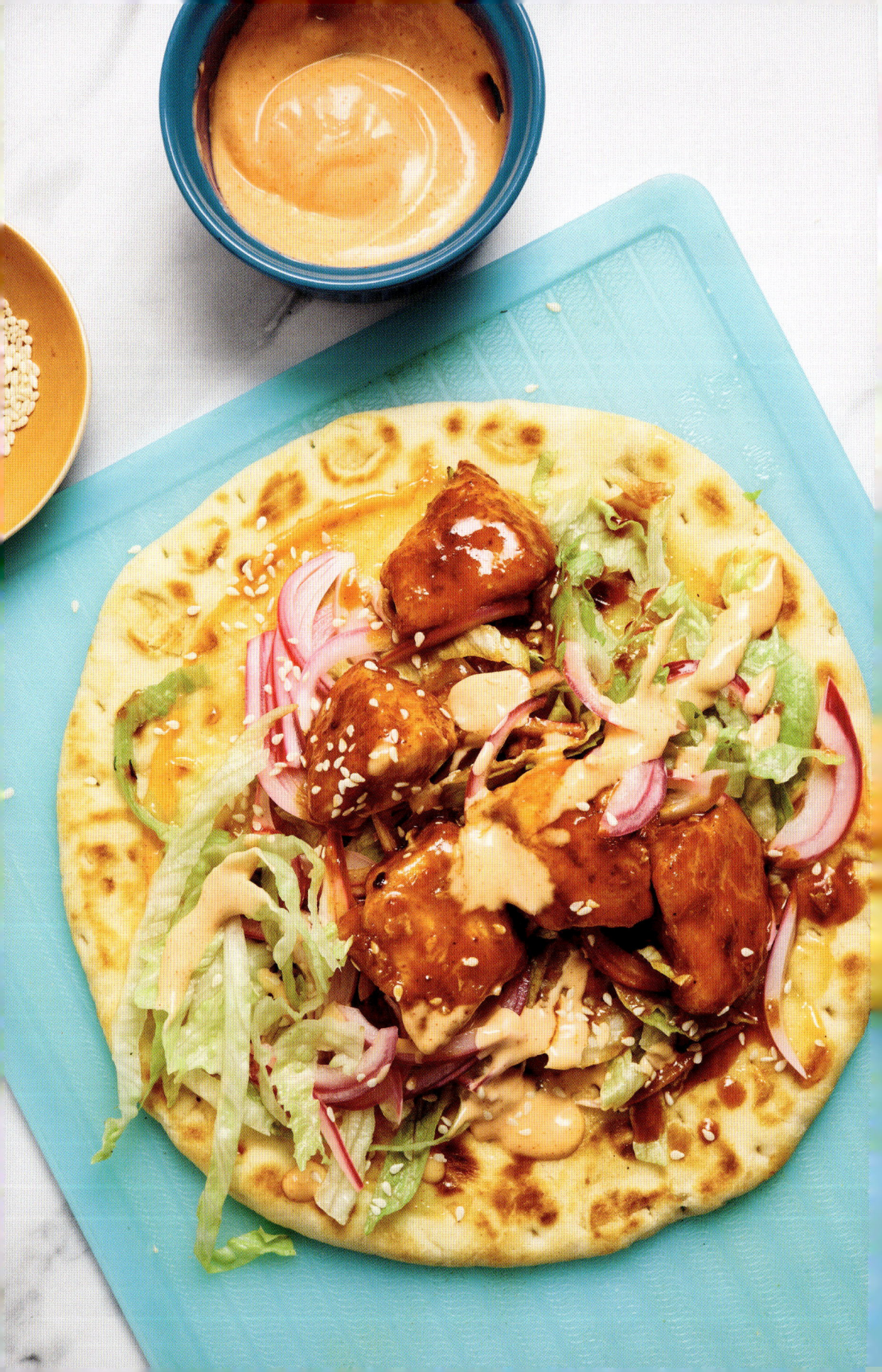

Sticky Gochujang Chicken Flatbreads

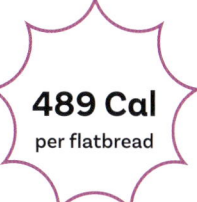

489 Cal per flatbread

Protein: 37.5g   Fat: 8.2g   Carbs: 63.5g

SERVES 2

Just when you think you've found your favourite flatbread recipe, another one enters your life, and this one is by far my favourite yet. I don't find the quantities of spice in this recipe that hot but if you are sensitive to spice, I recommend starting with a smaller amount of the gochujang paste!

Ingredients

200g skinless chicken breast, cut into 2.5cm cubes
¼ tsp paprika
¼ tsp garlic granules
1 tsp cornflour
Olive oil spray
1 small red onion, sliced
100ml distilled white vinegar
15g gochujang paste
30g runny honey
1 tbsp rice wine vinegar
½ tsp chopped garlic
2 tbsp light soy sauce
2 plain flatbreads
½ head of iceberg lettuce, finely shredded
1 tsp sesame seeds

Gochujang mayo sauce

50g lighter than light mayonnaise
½ tsp gochujang paste
½ tsp chopped garlic
1 tbsp rice vinegar

Method

- Season the chicken all over with the paprika and garlic granules. Once combined, mix in the cornflour.
- Heat a large pan over a high heat. Spray with a few pumps of olive oil spray, then add the chicken. Fry the chicken for 7–8 minutes, until cooked through.
- Put the onion into a bowl along with the distilled white vinegar and let it soak.
- In a bowl, mix together the sauce to go into the chicken by combining the gochujang paste, honey, rice wine vinegar, garlic and soy sauce, then set to one side.
- Mix together the ingredients for the gochujang mayo sauce and set to one side.
- By this point your chicken should be cooked, so heat the flatbreads according to the packet instructions.
- Pour the sauce for the chicken into the pan with the chicken, then turn the heat down to medium. After a minute, remove from the heat.
- Place the lettuce on top of each flatbread, along with the red onions, leaving the vinegar behind. Top with the chicken pieces, followed by the gochujang mayo sauce, and garnish with the sesame seeds.

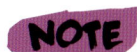

For all my recipes using gochujang paste, I'd suggest buying an authentic paste, which is usually found in the world food aisle in supermarkets.

Hot Honey Halloumi Tacos

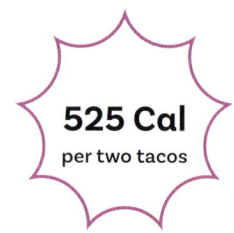

525 Cal per two tacos

| Protein: 30.9g | Fat: 22.8g | Carbs: 40.8g |

SERVES 2
(makes 4 mini tacos)

Hot honey was definitely made for halloumi – the balance between sweet and salt is really delicious. This recipe calls for the halloumi to be served in some mini tortillas along with crispy lettuce, a homemade garlic sauce, and pomegranate seeds for a burst of freshness. If you prefer a bit of a bite to your tacos, place them in a hot dry pan for 45 seconds on each side.

Ingredients

200g reduced-fat halloumi, sliced
1 tsp smoked paprika
1 tsp garlic granules
2 tsp cornflour
Olive oil spray
30g runny honey
1 tsp hot sauce
4 mini tortilla wraps
75g sweet crispy salad leaves
20g pomegranate seeds
A few chilli flakes, to garnish (optional)

Garlic sauce
40g fat-free Greek yoghurt
¼ tsp garlic granules
1 tsp distilled white vinegar
½ tsp dried parsley

Method

- Start by patting the halloumi dry with kitchen paper. Season on both sides with the smoked paprika and garlic granules and rub in thoroughly.
- Sprinkle over the cornflour on both sides and rub in thoroughly.
- Heat a large frying pan over a medium-high heat. Spray with a few pumps of olive oil before adding the halloumi, ensuring there is space around each piece.
- Leave undisturbed for 2 minutes before flipping and cooking for a further 2 minutes.
- While the halloumi cooks, in a small bowl mix together the honey and hot sauce.
- Make the garlic sauce by mixing all the ingredients in a separate bowl and set to one side.
- Once you have flipped the halloumi for the final time, pour in the hot honey sauce. Leave over a medium-low heat for a minute before flipping for a final minute.
- Warm the tortilla wraps slightly in the microwave on high for 10-15 seconds.
- Top the wraps with the crispy salad leaves, followed by the halloumi. Drizzle over the garlic sauce, along with any honey sauce from the halloumi pan, then scatter with the pomegranate seeds, and the chilli flakes if using.

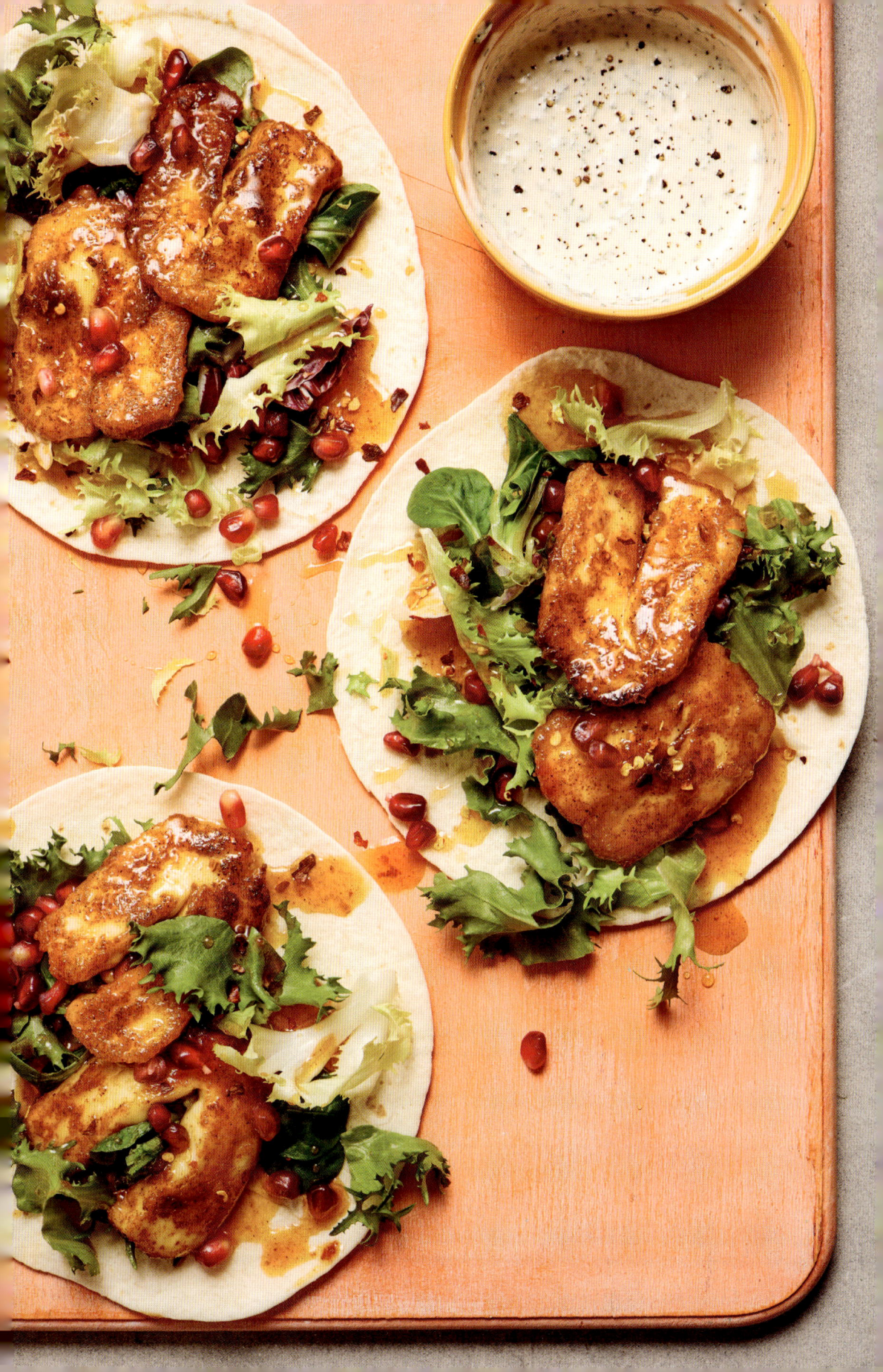

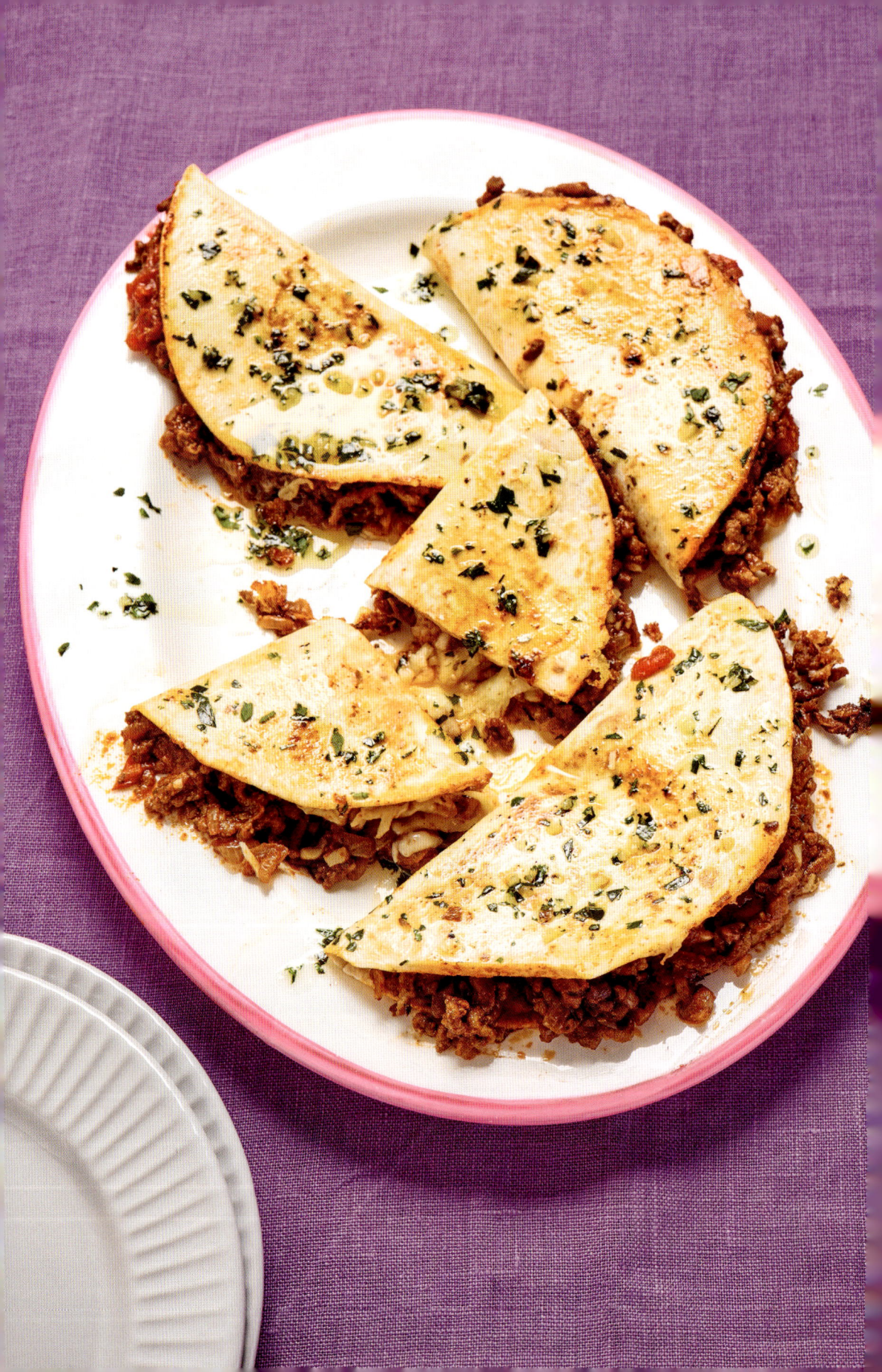

Garlic Butter Chilli Beef Tacos

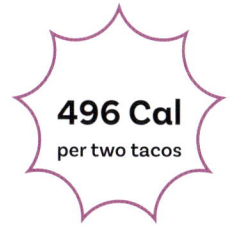

496 Cal per two tacos

Protein: 43.5g **Fat: 26.4g** **Carbs: 29.3g**

SERVES 2
(makes 4 mini tacos)

Taco Tuesday is calling and, oh boy, are these tacos a banger. This recipe went viral on my social media and I can understand why. A quick chilli beef is whipped up and tucked into crispy mini wraps with cheddar and a brush of garlic butter for a taco like no other. I usually have these with a nice side salad, but you can serve them with Mexican rice or some nachos if you want to.

Ingredients

Olive oil spray
1 white onion, diced
2 tsp chopped garlic
200g lean beef mince
½ tbsp mild chilli powder
1 tsp paprika
1 tsp ground cumin
1 tsp ground coriander
1 tsp mixed herbs
1 beef stock cube, crumbled
100ml water
1 tbsp tomato purée
1 tsp granulated sweetener
100g chopped tomatoes
4 mini tortilla wraps
60g reduced-fat cheddar, grated
10g light butter
2 sprigs of fresh coriander, chopped
Salt and pepper

Method

- Start by spraying a large frying pan with a few pumps of olive oil spray. Fry the onion for a minute before adding 1 teaspoon of the garlic and frying for a further minute.
- Add the beef mince to the same pan and fry for 3-4 minutes, until slightly brown.
- Add the chilli powder, paprika, cumin, coriander, mixed herbs and some salt and pepper. Mix in well before adding the crumbled stock cube, water, tomato purée, sweetener and chopped tomatoes. Leave to simmer over a medium-high heat.
- Meanwhile, heat a large frying pan over a medium heat. Add each mini wrap to the pan and fry for 45-60 seconds each side, until slightly toasted.
- Remove from the pan and top each wrap with the cheddar, then with the chilli beef. Fold in half and return to the pan. Fry for 2 minutes on each side until the cheese has melted and the outside of the wraps is slightly crispy.
- While the wraps cook, Put the butter and remaining teaspoon of chopped garlic into a microwavable bowl. Blast in the microwave on medium for 15 seconds until melted, then stir through half of the fresh coriander.
- Brush the garlic butter over the top of the tacos and remove from the pan. Scatter over the remaining coriander and serve.

Crispy Orange Chicken

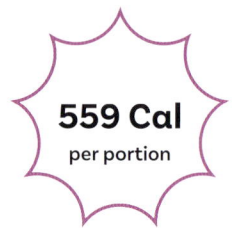

559 Cal per portion

| Protein: 43.4g | Fat: 4.9g | Carbs: 84.2g |

SERVES 2

 AF

Crispy chicken is coated in a delicious sweet and tangy orange sauce. You might be thinking that combination is a bit strange if you haven't tried it before, but it seriously tastes amazing, and this is the perfect recipe for a weekend fakeaway. You can serve this with rice as listed or over noodles if you prefer, and if you like a kick to your dishes, add some chopped red chilli for a spicy version.

Ingredients

1 × 125g packet of boil-in-the-bag rice
250g skinless chicken breast, cut into 2.5cm cubes
1 tsp garlic granules
½ tsp paprika
30g egg white
35g cornflour
Neutral cooking spray
Salt and pepper
1 spring onion, sliced, to garnish
½ tsp sesame seeds, to garnish

Sauce
100ml freshly squeezed orange juice
25ml light soy sauce
25ml dark soy sauce
1 tbsp brown sugar
1 tsp cornflour
Zest of 1 orange
2 tsp chopped garlic
1 tsp chopped ginger

Method

- Start by cooking the rice according to the packet instructions.
- Put the chicken into a bowl. Season with a pinch of salt and pepper along with the garlic granules and paprika before mixing in the egg white.
- Dip each piece of chicken into the cornflour, shaking off any excess. Transfer to the air fryer basket, spray with a few pumps of cooking spray and cook for 14 minutes at 195ºC. (Alternatively, transfer to a hot frying pan sprayed with neutral cooking spray and cook over a high heat for 8–10 minutes.)
- While the chicken cooks, make up the sauce by mixing all the ingredients except the garlic and ginger in a bowl.
- When there are 5 minutes left of the chicken cooking time, heat a small pan over a medium heat and add the garlic and ginger. Fry for 1 minute, until aromatic, then pour in the sauce.
- Leave the sauce to thicken while the chicken finishes cooking. If necessary, you can turn up the heat slightly to help thicken it further.
- Once the chicken has cooked and the sauce has reduced, add the chicken to the sauce, stirring to coat.
- Serve the cooked rice with the chicken on top, drizzling over any remaining sauce. Garnish with the sliced spring onion and the sesame seeds.

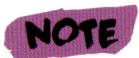

You can add honey to the sauce to sweeten it, if you like.

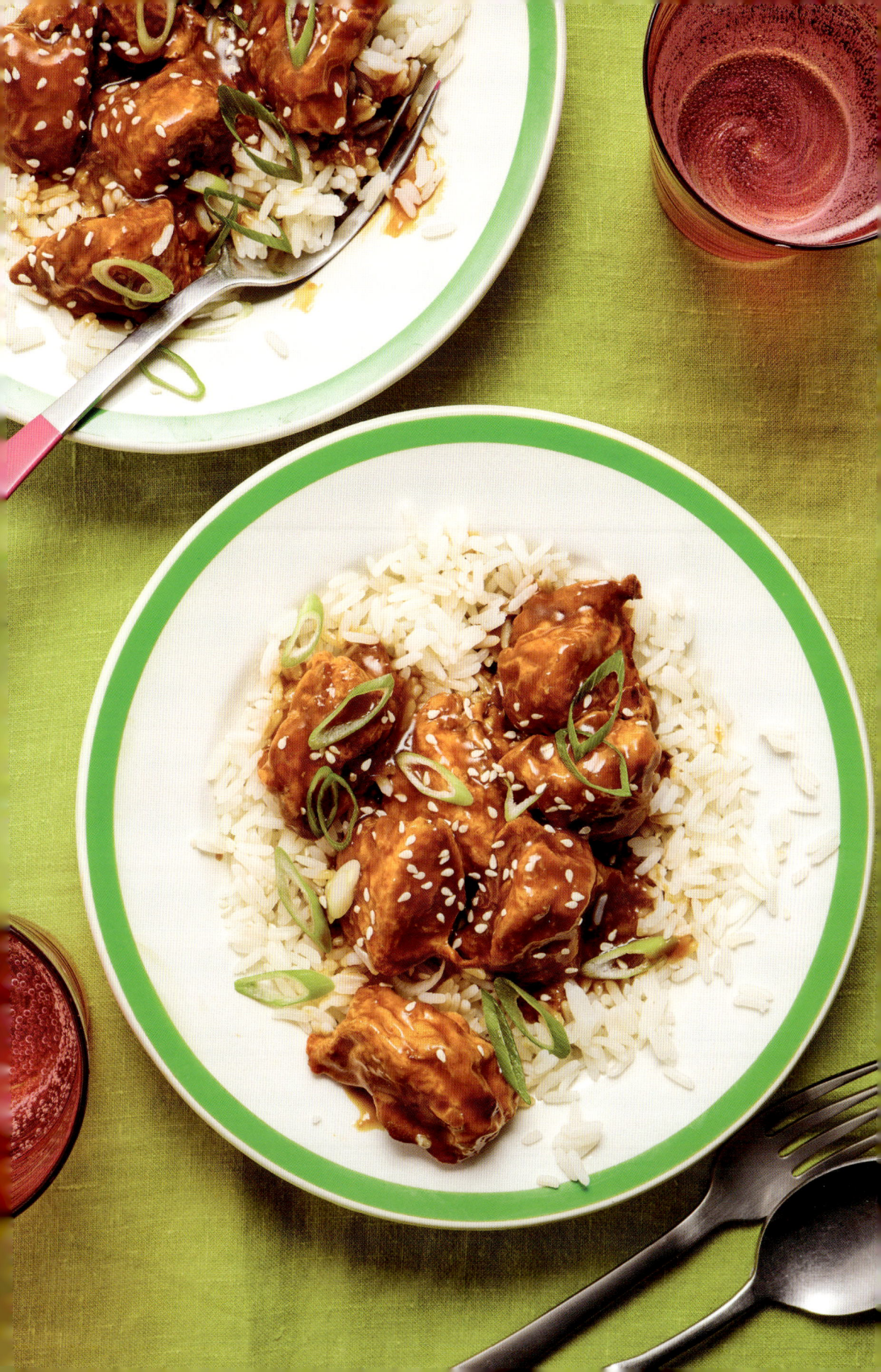

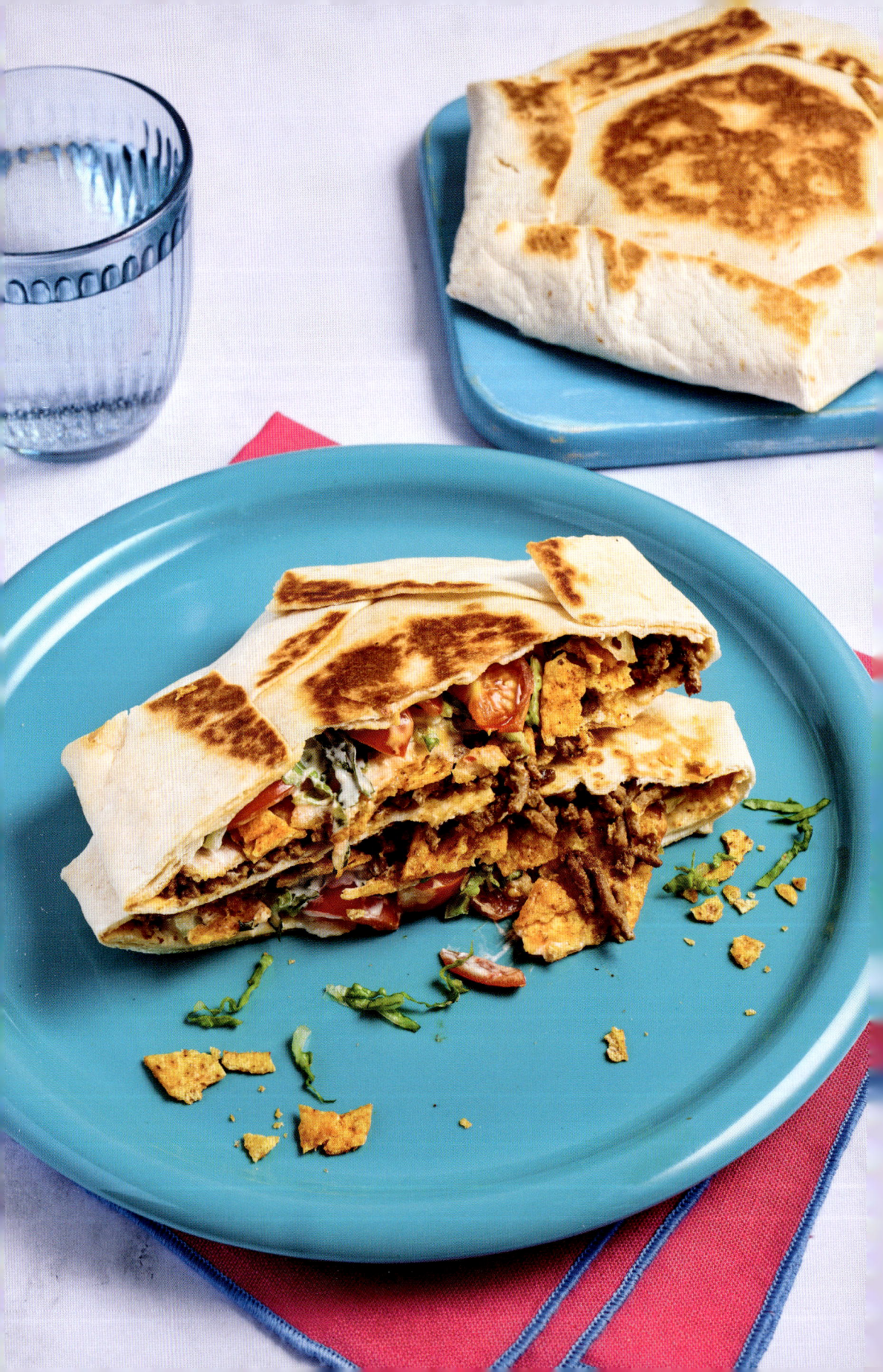

Crunchwrap Supreme

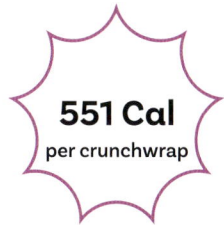

551 Cal per crunchwrap

Protein: 32.3g **Fat: 16.8g** **Carbs: 63.2g**

MAKES 2

If you haven't yet tried a Crunchwrap Supreme, your mind is about to be blown. Beef is layered on a wrap with nacho cheese dip, crunchy tortilla chips, Greek yoghurt, lettuce and tomatoes. Seriously, every single bite is super addictive.

Ingredients

Olive oil spray
200g lean beef mince
2 tbsp taco seasoning
80ml water
2 tortilla wraps
50g nacho cheese dip
20g tortilla chips
40g fat-free Greek yoghurt
2 handfuls of shredded lettuce
80g cherry tomatoes, quartered
2 mini tortilla wraps

Method

- Spray a frying pan with olive oil spray and place over a high heat. Add the beef mince and fry for a couple of minutes. When almost browned, add the taco seasoning and fry for a further minute.
- Pour in the water and leave to reduce over a high heat. Once the sauce has reduced and feels thick, turn off the heat but leave the pan on the hob.
- Place a large, clean, dry frying pan with no oil over a medium heat.
- In the centre of each larger tortilla wrap, spread the nacho cheese dip equally in a circle shape. Top with the cooked beef mince, then the tortilla chips. Dollop the Greek yoghurt on top, followed by the shredded lettuce and tomatoes.
- Place the mini wraps over the top of the filling, pressing down slightly. Fold the edges of the large tortillas towards the centre, creating pleats as you go. Quickly flip over and place the wraps pleat-side down in the pan (you may need to cook each wrap separately, depending on the size of your pan).
- Leave the wraps pleat-side down for 2 minutes before flipping and cooking for a further minute.
- Remove from the heat and serve.

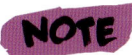

If you struggle to fold wraps, blast them in the microwave on medium for 10–15 seconds first. If you don't want to buy two lots of wraps, simply grab your large tortillas and draw a mini circle shape to create mini tortillas using a cereal bowl as a guide.

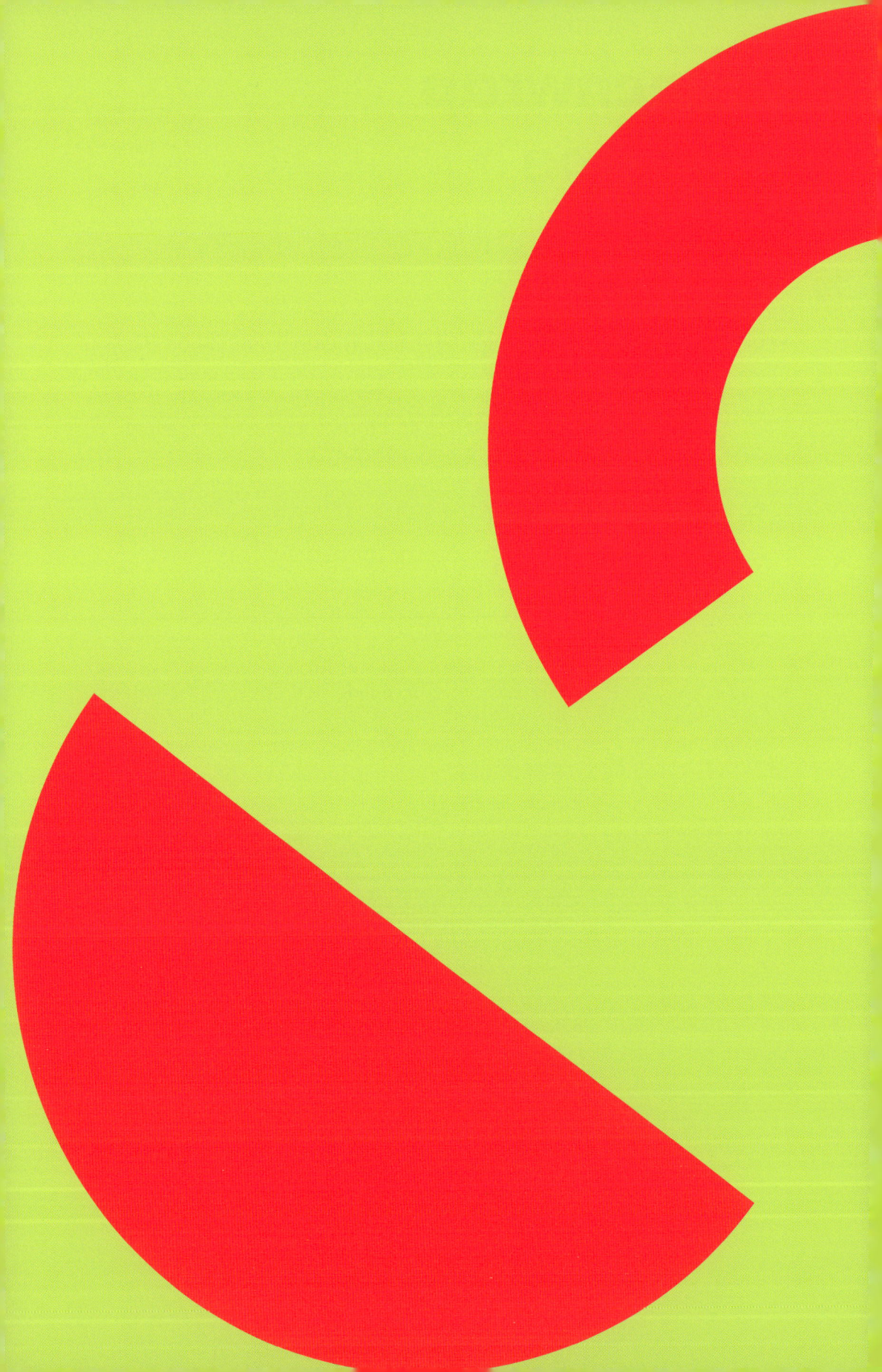

Seven

POP IT IN THE PAN

Chicken Gravy Stuffing Baguettes

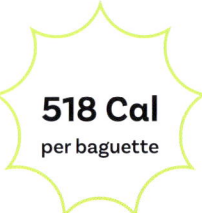

518 Cal per baguette

| Protein: 39.8g | Fat: 5.1g | Carbs: 71.6g |

MAKES 2

Even if you're pressed for time, you can still savour some comfort food. These baguettes are quick to prepare as everything is cooked in a single pan. Seasoned chicken pieces are combined with onion, stuffing and gravy, then stuffed into a crispy baguette for a delicious bite. Pair them with steamed vegetables or some roast potatoes.

Ingredients

Olive oil spray

200g skinless chicken breast, cut into 2.5cm cubes

1 tsp garlic granules

1 tsp onion granules

25g sage and onion stuffing mix

300ml hot water

35g chicken gravy granules

1 white onion, diced

2 baguettes, sliced (100g each)

Salt and pepper

A few sprigs of fresh parsley, chopped, to garnish

Method

- Start by spraying a large frying pan with olive oil spray and heating over a medium-high heat.

- In a bowl, season the chicken pieces with the garlic granules, onion granules and some salt and pepper. Rub the seasonings in thoroughly before transferring the chicken to the pan. Cook over a high heat for 8 minutes, making sure to keep moving the chicken around to brown it evenly.

- Meanwhile, in a bowl add the stuffing mix followed by 50ml of the water. Mix in well until the water has disappeared. Leave to stand.

- Next, put the gravy granules into a jug along with the remaining 250ml of water, mix to combine. If needed, thin out to your desired consistency.

- Once the 8 minutes has elapsed, turn the heat under the chicken pan down to medium and add the onion, cooking for a couple of minutes until soft.

- When the onion is soft, add the stuffing, breaking into smaller pieces, along with three quarters of the gravy, reserving the rest to serve. Leave over the heat for a minute until everything is combined.

- Pack the chicken and stuffing mix into the baguettes, garnishing with the fresh parsley. Serve with the remaining gravy for dunking.

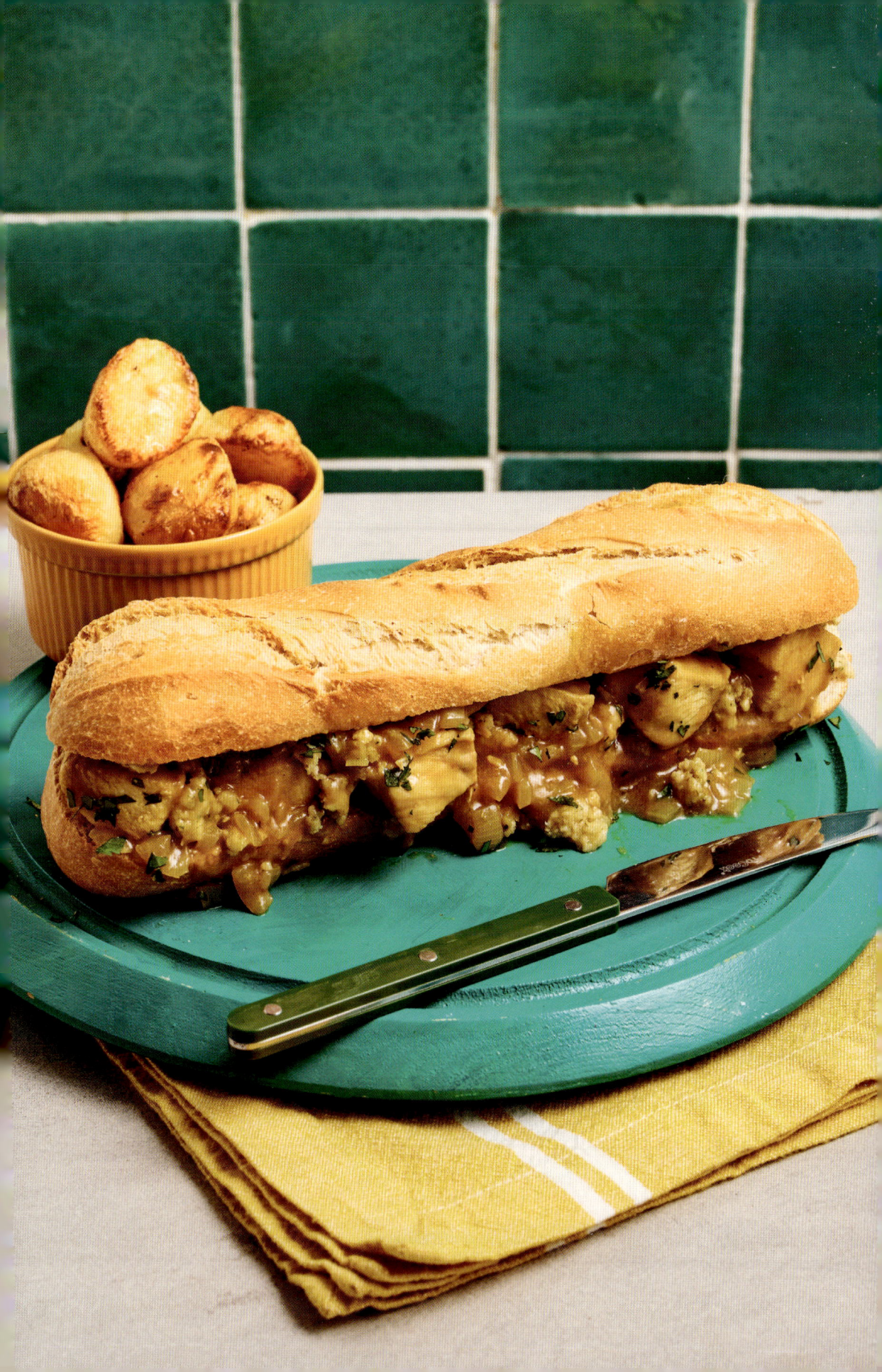

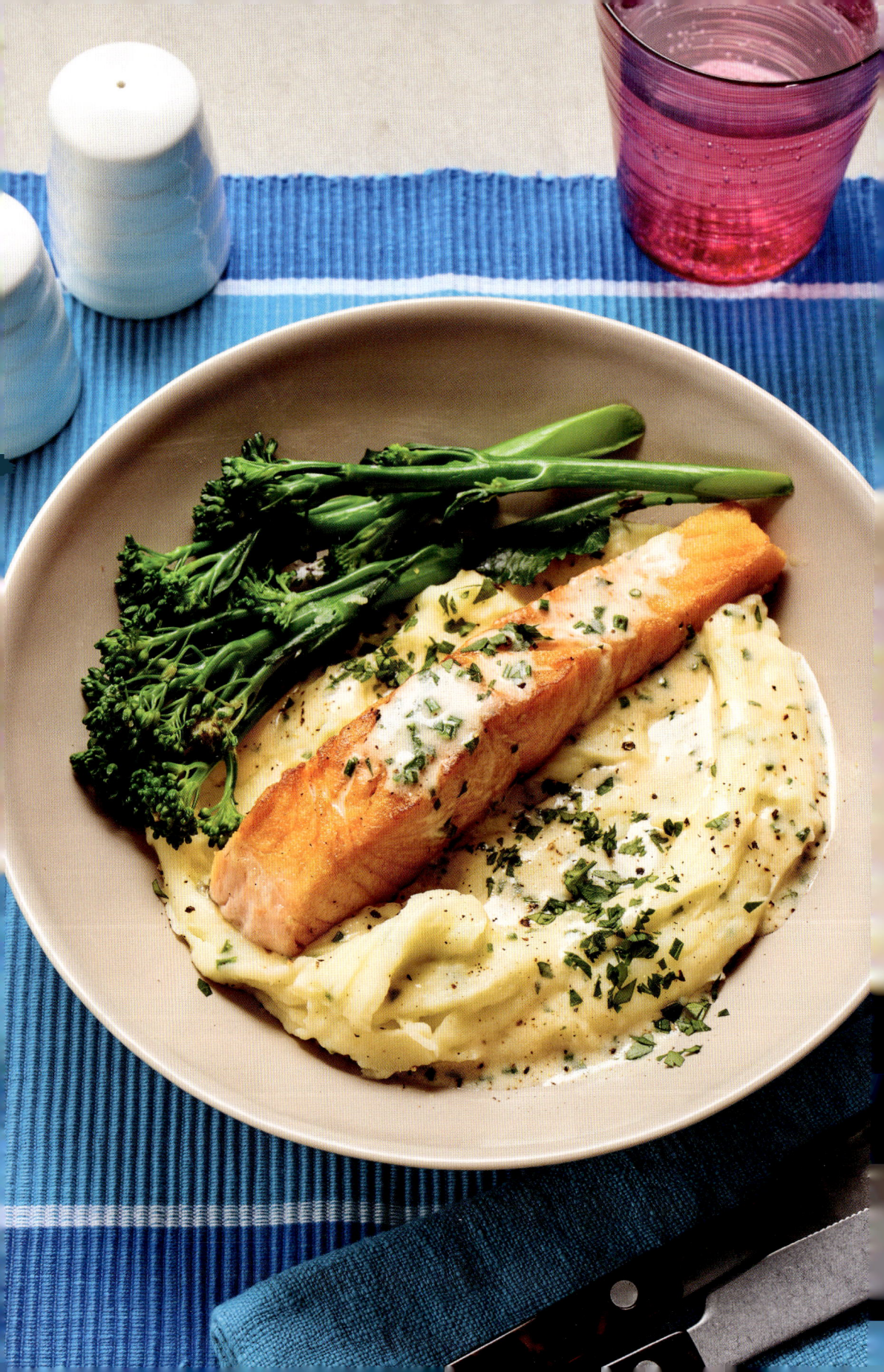

Cheesy Herby Salmon and Mash

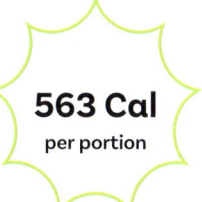

563 Cal per portion

Protein: 38.8g **Fat: 23g** **Carbs: 44.3g**

SERVES 2

The sauce in this recipe will have you wanting to lick the pan clean. It is that good. Made up with garlic, cream cheese, cheddar and Parmesan with parsley and chives to really pack a punch. If you're anti-fish, this recipe can also be made with chicken and even steak.

Ingredients

500g Maris Piper potatoes, peeled and cut into small cubes
2 salmon fillets (260g in total)
Olive oil spray
1 tsp chopped garlic
30g light cream cheese
100ml chicken stock
30g reduced-fat cheddar, grated
15g Parmesan, grated
3 sprigs of fresh parsley, chopped
4 chives, chopped
50ml water
15g light butter
75ml semi-skimmed milk
Salt and pepper

Method

- Start by placing the potatoes in a large pan of salted boiling water. Cook for 14-15 minutes over a high heat until tender when pierced with a fork.
- Season both sides of the salmon with salt and pepper.
- Spray a large pan with a few pumps of olive oil spray. Add the salmon to the pan and cook for 3 minutes before turning for a further 2 minutes. Remove from the pan and set to one side.
- Turn down the heat, then add the garlic, cream cheese and chicken stock. Stir to combine and leave over a medium heat for 2 minutes.
- Next, stir through the cheddar and Parmesan before adding three quarters of the parsley, three quarters of the chopped chives and a pinch of salt and pepper.
- Use the water to loosen the sauce. If the sauce turns too thick, add a little more water to achieve your desired consistency. Turn the heat down low.
- Once the potatoes are cooked, drain and season with salt and pepper. Add the butter and milk along with the rest of the chives. Mash together using a potato masher or, if you have one, an electric hand whisk.
- Serve the mashed potatoes with the salmon on top. Drizzle over the cream sauce and garnish with the remaining parsley.

Deconstructed Enchiladas

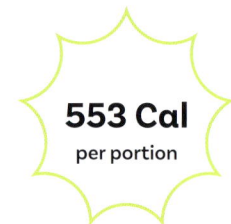

553 Cal per portion

Protein: 45g **Fat: 16g** **Carbs: 51.4g**

SERVES 2

One of my favourite Mexican dishes is enchiladas. This is a one-pan version and the flavours are guaranteed to make your eyes roll into the back of your head; it truly is that good. It's a great way to use up any leftover stale wraps you have floating in the cupboard, but, if you like a bit more bite to your meal, opt for corn tortillas instead. If you can't find enchilada sauce or fancy a change, fajita or chilli cooking sauce also works well here.

Ingredients

Olive oil spray
1 red onion, diced
1 red pepper, diced
1 tsp chopped garlic
200g extra lean beef mince
1 tbsp taco seasoning
200g enchilada sauce
100ml water
1 tsp chipotle paste
1 tsp lime juice
2 tortillas
40g reduced-fat cheddar, grated
20g Red Leicester, grated
3 sprigs of fresh coriander, chopped
A few jalapeños, to garnish (optional)

Method

- Heat a medium frying pan over a medium-high heat and spray with olive oil spray.
- Add the red onion and red pepper and fry for 2 minutes until slightly soft, then add the garlic for a further minute.
- Add the beef mince, breaking it up into smaller pieces, and continue to cook for 3 minutes before adding in the taco seasoning. Mix well, then add the enchilada sauce, water, chipotle paste and lime juice.
- While the sauce thickens, cut the tortillas into 3cm strips and then cut the strips again in half.
- Add the cut tortillas to the pan, toss the tortillas to ensure they are in the sauce and spread out evenly.
- Once evenly distributed, scatter both grated cheeses on top. Cover the pan for 2-3 minutes until the cheese has melted and is bubbling.
- Serve with the fresh coriander, and the jalapeños if using.

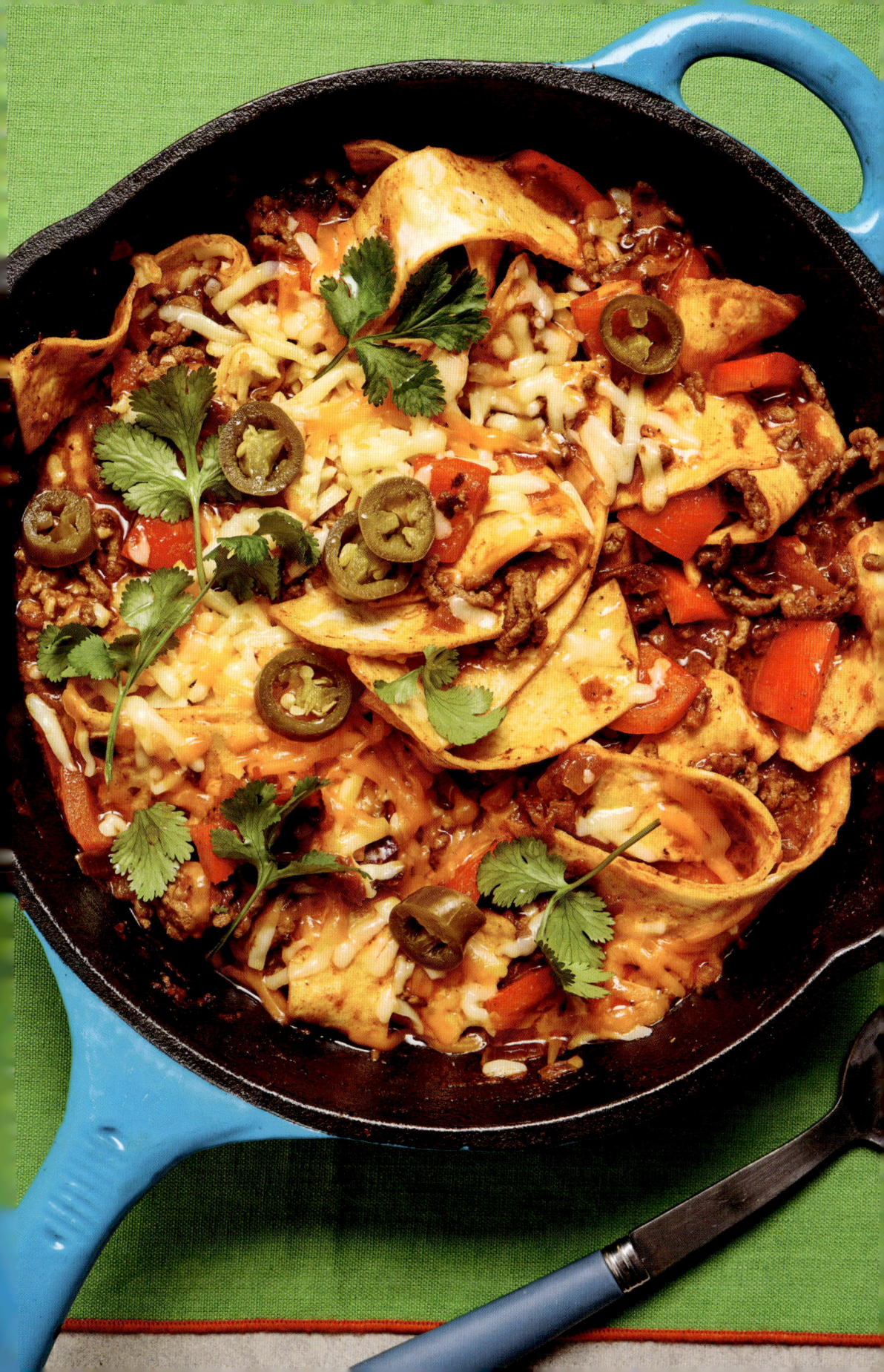

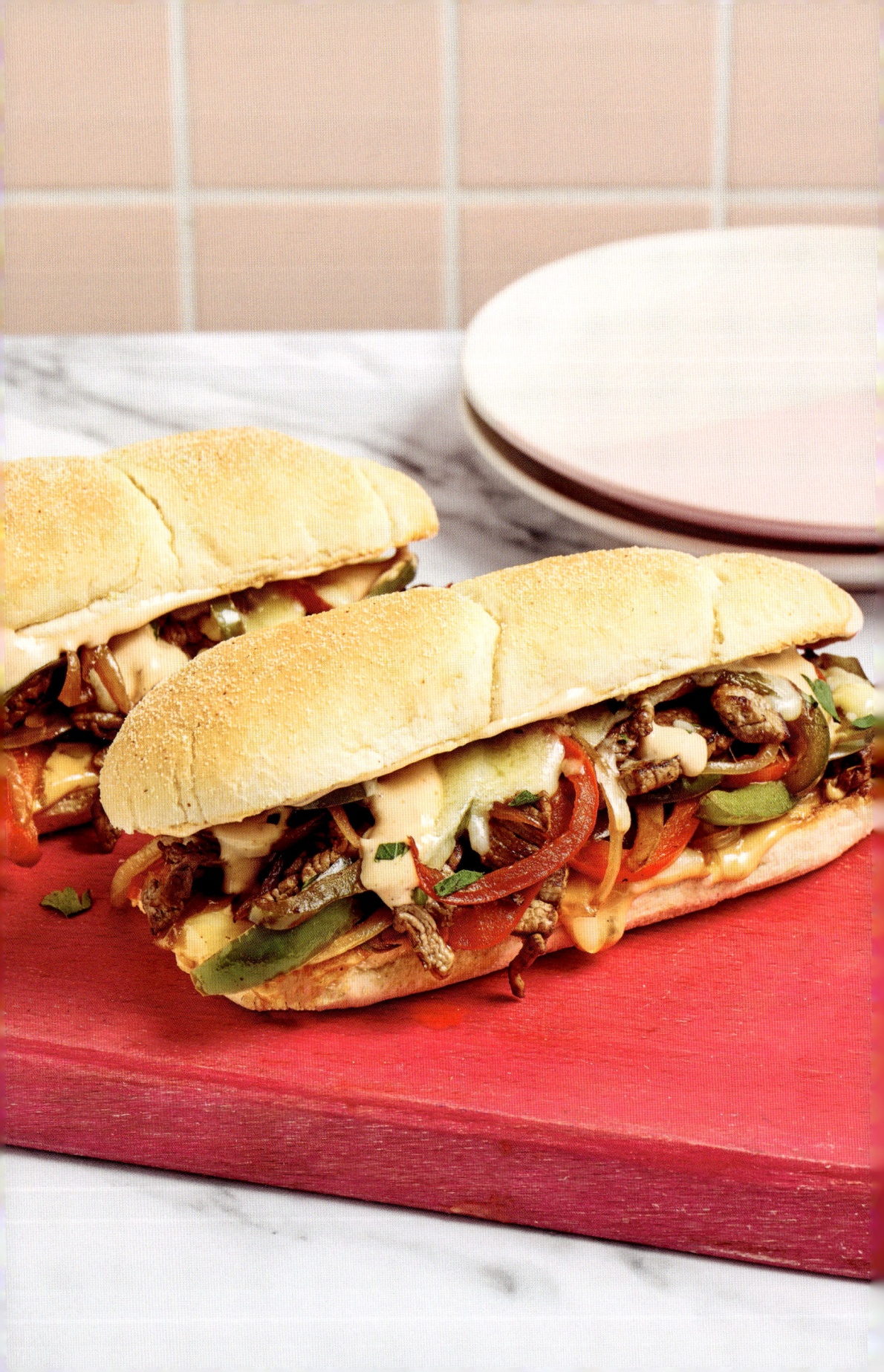

Chipotle Cheesesteak Sub

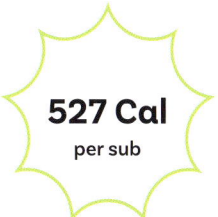

527 Cal per sub

Protein: 42.4g **Fat: 11.9g** **Carbs: 59.2g**

SERVES 2

This recipe puts a gorgeous twist on the classic Philly. Peppers and onion are fried until soft, then tossed with thinly sliced steak and piled into a sub roll with plenty of cheese and a gorgeous chipotle sauce. It's a certified banger.

Ingredients

200g rump steak
Olive oil spray
1 tsp chopped garlic
1 white onion, thinly sliced
1 small red pepper, thinly sliced
1 small green pepper, thinly sliced
1 tbsp Worcestershire sauce
40g lighter than light mayonnaise
½ tsp garlic granules
1 tsp chipotle paste
3 tbsp hot water
2 sub rolls
60g reduced-fat cheddar, grated
Salt
2 sprigs of fresh parsley, chopped, to garnish

Method

- Preheat the grill to medium.
- Start by thinly slicing the steak against the grain.
- Spray a large frying pan with a few pumps of olive oil spray, then add the chopped garlic, onion and peppers. Fry over a high heat for 2 minutes until softened, then add in the Worcestershire sauce for a further minute.
- Meanwhile, mix the mayonnaise, garlic granules, chipotle paste and a pinch of salt, then add the hot water and mix well until combined.
- Remove the veggies from the pan, add the steak and cook for a minute, then toss and cook for a further 30 seconds. Note that you want it slightly underdone before melting the cheese.
- Return the veggies to the pan and toss to combine.
- Slice the sub rolls in half and place under a hot grill for 30-60 seconds until lightly toasted.
- Top the bottom halves of each roll with half of the chipotle sauce and half of the cheddar, followed by the steak and veggies, followed by the remaining cheddar.
- Place back under the grill for a couple of minutes until the cheese has melted, then cover with the top halves of the rolls.
- Serve with the remaining sauce drizzled over and garnished with the parsley.

Pesto Chicken and Broccoli Rice

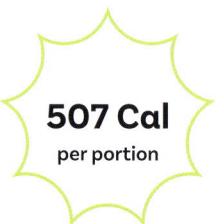

507 Cal per portion

Protein: 41.8g **Fat: 11.4g** **Carbs: 55.4g**

SERVES 2

This is such a feel-good recipe. Pesto is the star of the show in this cream cheese sauce, packed with cherry tomatoes for an added burst of flavour. Chopping broccoli up into rice is a brilliant way to add more volume to your meals, plus it's a great hack for any fussy eaters.

Ingredients

2 × 62.5g packets of boil-in-the-bag long-grain rice

150g broccoli florets

200g skinless chicken breast, cut into 2.5cm cubes

Olive oil spray

1 tsp chopped garlic

100g cherry tomatoes, quartered

1 chicken stock cube, crumbled

40g reduced-fat green pesto

60g light cream cheese

100ml water

10g Parmesan, grated

Salt and pepper

A few basil leaves, torn, to garnish

Method

- Start by cooking the rice according to the packet instructions, which should take around 15 minutes. When there are 7 minutes remaining on the cooking time, add the broccoli to the same pan.

- Next, season the chicken with salt and pepper. Spray a large frying pan with a few pumps of olive oil spray. Add the chicken to the pan, along with the garlic. Fry over a high heat for 4 minutes before adding the tomatoes. Continue to fry until the chicken is cooked through.

- Once the chicken has cooked, add the stock cube, pesto, cream cheese and water to the pan. Mix well and leave over a medium heat.

- When the rice has cooked, remove the rice bags and strain the broccoli, before using a spatula to crush down the pieces of broccoli into small bits. Cut the bags of rice open and combine with the broccoli.

- Stir the Parmesan into the pesto sauce and remove from the heat.

- Serve the broccoli rice topped with the pesto chicken and garnished with the basil leaves.

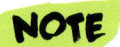

This recipe is suitable for meal prep. Double the quantities and allow to cool completely before storing in an airtight container. Keep in the fridge for up to three days.

Chicken Parm Pasta

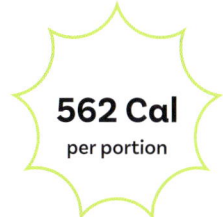

562 Cal per portion

Protein: 43.8g | Fat: 15.9g | Carbs: 54.8g

SERVES 2

All the amazing flavours of a chicken parm but in pasta form. Don't worry, we're not missing out the breadcrumbs – instead they're pan fried in some butter and sprinkled over the top for that perfect golden crunch.

Ingredients

120g dried pasta

200g skinless chicken breast, cut into 2.5cm cubes

½ tsp garlic granules

Olive oil spray

10g light butter

10g panko breadcrumbs

1 white onion, diced

1½ tsp chopped garlic

1½ tsp Italian herb seasoning

1 tbsp tomato purée

150g good-quality passata

1 chicken stock cube, crumbled

120ml reduced-fat single cream alternative (I use Elmlea; see NOTE), or you can sub for reduced-fat crème fraîche

20g Parmesan, grated

Salt and pepper

A few sprigs of fresh parsley, chopped, to garnish

Method

- Start by cooking the pasta in boiling salted water according to the packet instructions.
- Season the chicken with salt, pepper and the garlic granules. Spray a large frying pan with a few pumps of olive oil spray. Over a high heat, fry the chicken for 7 minutes or so, until golden.
- While the chicken cooks, heat a separate pan over a medium heat. Add the butter, leave to melt, then add the breadcrumbs. Cook for 3 minutes, moving the crumbs around in the pan, until golden, then turn off the heat but leave on the stove to keep warm.
- Once the chicken is golden, add the onion followed by the garlic and cook for 1 minute. Next, add the herb seasoning, salt and pepper to taste, followed by the tomato purée, passata and stock cube and mix well for 1 minute. Turn down the heat and pour in the cream.
- Leave the sauce to thicken while you drain the pasta, reserving 50ml of the pasta water.
- Add the pasta to the sauce, along with half the Parmesan. Mix well, stirring through the reserved pasta water as well.
- Serve the pasta and top with the remaining Parmesan, followed by the golden breadcrumbs and the parsley.

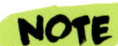

You can use 60ml single cream and 60ml semi-skimmed milk in place of the cream alternative, ensuring the heat is turned down low so that the sauce doesn't split.

Saucy Korean-Style Chicken with Brown Rice

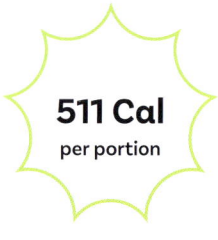

511 Cal per portion

Protein: 34.7g   Fat: 10.2g   Carbs: 66.4g

SERVES 2

The sauce in this recipe will have you licking the bowl afterwards, it genuinely is that good. The main components are gochujang paste, honey and soy sauce – these create a glaze for the crispy pan-fried bites of chicken. Pack out this meal with some Tenderstem broccoli, grated carrot or pak choi.

Ingredients

- 10ml sesame oil
- 200g skinless chicken breast, cut into 2.5cm cubes
- ½ tsp smoked paprika
- ½ tsp garlic granules
- 1 tsp soy sauce
- 20g egg white
- 25g cornflour
- 1 × 250g packet of brown microwave rice
- 2 spring onions, sliced, to garnish
- ½ tsp sesame seeds, to garnish

Sauce
- 20g gochujang paste
- 30g runny honey
- 30ml light soy sauce
- 1 tsp chopped garlic
- 1 tsp ginger purée
- 1 tsp brown sugar

Method

- Start by putting the sesame oil into a large frying pan over a medium-high heat.
- In a bowl, season the chicken with the smoked paprika and garlic granules. Add the soy sauce and egg white and mix well.
- Put the cornflour into a separate bowl. Dip each piece of chicken into the cornflour, shaking off any excess. Once all the pieces are coated, transfer them to the hot pan. Fry for 10 minutes, continuously moving the chicken around the pan for an even crispness.
- Meanwhile, in a bowl, mix together the sauce ingredients.
- Once the chicken is evenly crispy and cooked through, take the pan off the heat. Pour in the sauce ingredients, mix well and place the pan back on a low heat.
- Microwave the rice according to the packet instructions.
- Serve the cooked rice in a bowl with the chicken alongside and drizzle over the sauce. Garnish with the spring onions and sesame seeds.

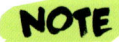

For extra crispy chicken, at step 3 you can cook the chicken in the air fryer for 15 minutes at 190°C. For all my recipes using gochujang paste, I really recommend buying an authentic paste, which is usually found in the world food aisle in supermarkets.

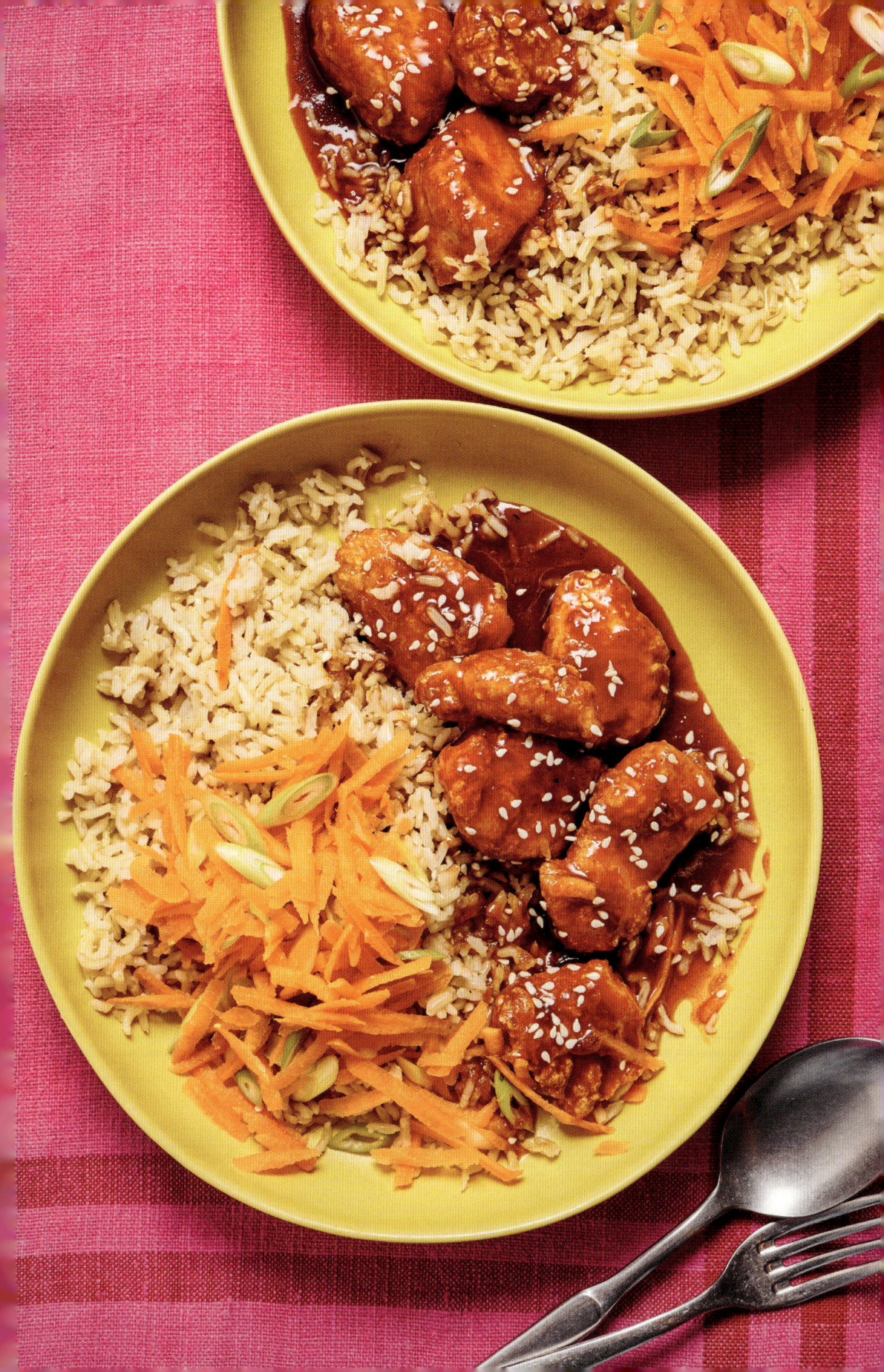

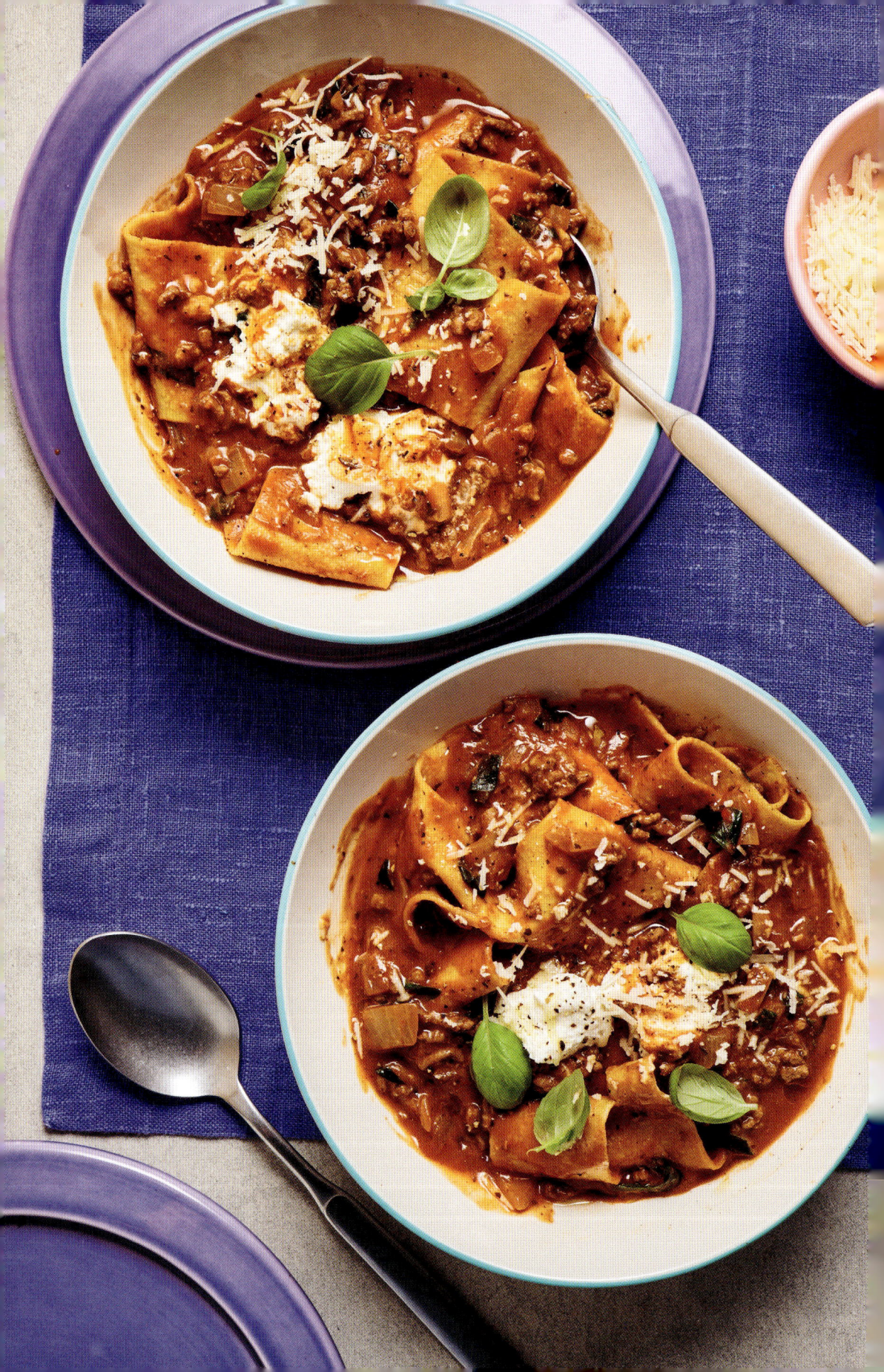

Lasagne Soup

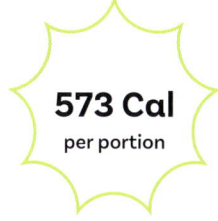

573 Cal per portion

| Protein: 52.2g | Fat: 18.45g | Carbs: 44.15g |

SERVES 2

If you're in serious need of some comfort food, make this recipe; it's how I imagine a hug from food would feel like. If you don't like ricotta, you can omit this; the soup will taste just as good without it! You can also easily double it and store it in the fridge for up to four days as meal prep.

Ingredients

Olive oil spray
1 white onion, diced
1 heaped tsp chopped garlic
250g lean beef mince
1 tsp Italian herb seasoning
1 tsp smoked paprika
1 tsp dried oregano
1 tbsp tomato purée
1 tsp granulated sweetener (optional)
300g good-quality passata
400ml hot beef stock made with 2 cubes
50ml reduced-fat single cream alternative (I use Elmlea; you could use milk left to come to room temperature instead)
5 fresh egg lasagne sheets (25g per sheet)
2 handfuls of spinach, chopped
50g ricotta
40g mozzarella, grated
5g Parmesan, grated
Salt and pepper
A few fresh basil leaves, to garnish

Method

- Start by spraying a large pan with olive oil spray. Over a high heat fry the onion for 1 minute, until slightly soft, then add the garlic for 30 seconds.

- Next, add the beef, continuing to cook over a high heat for 3–4 minutes until almost browned. Then turn down the heat slightly while you add the seasonings – the Italian herb seasoning, smoked paprika and oregano along with some salt and pepper to taste. Mix into the meat.

- Once the seasonings are combined, add the tomato purée, sweetener, if using, passata, beef stock and cream. Bring to a high heat and cook for a minute.

- While the sauce is boiling, slice the lasagne sheets in half and then half again. Add them to the pan, mixing well to ensure they are covered in the liquid. Leave over a medium heat for 3 minutes or so, by which time they should start to soften.

- Add the chopped spinach and cook for a further 2 minutes.

- While the spinach wilts, in a bowl, season the ricotta with salt and pepper, then whisk together and set to one side. Once the spinach has wilted, stir through the grated mozzarella.

- Remove the pan from the heat. Dollop the ricotta on top of the lasagne, then sprinkle with the Parmesan and garnish with fresh basil leaves.

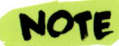

If you like your soup to be more 'brothy', add an extra 100ml of water.

Gochujang Chicken Pasta

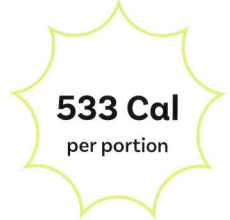

533 Cal per portion

Protein: 43.9g | Fat: 14.2g | Carbs: 51.8g

SERVES 2

This is one of those fusion dishes you can't believe tastes as good as it does. I really recommend ensuring you get hold of authentic Korean gochujang paste rather than supermarket-own brands, as the taste does vary greatly. You can usually find it in the world food aisle. Start with the listed amount and increase as needed to suit your spice palate.

Ingredients

200g skinless chicken breast, cut into 2.5cm cubes
1 tsp onion granules
1 tsp garlic granules
½ tsp paprika
Olive oil spray
120g dried rigatoni
1 shallot, finely diced
2 tsp chopped garlic
15g gochujang paste (I use Daesang)
1 tbsp tomato purée
120ml reduced-fat single cream alternative (I use Elmlea; see NOTE)
30g Parmesan, grated
Salt and pepper
½ tsp chilli flakes, to garnish (optional)
A few sprigs of fresh parsley, chopped, to garnish

Method

- Start by seasoning the chicken with the onion granules, garlic granules and paprika, along with a pinch of salt and pepper.
- Spray a large frying pan with a few pumps of olive oil spray. Fry the chicken over a high heat for 8 minutes.
- While the chicken cooks, put the pasta in a large pan of boiling salted water and cook according to the packet instructions.
- Add the shallot and garlic to the chicken and fry for 1 minute. Remove the pan from the heat, while you add the gochujang paste, tomato purée and cream. Mix well to combine and leave over a low heat until the pasta is cooked.
- Once the pasta is cooked, drain, reserving 100ml of the water, and set to one side.
- Add the reserved pasta water to the sauce along with 20g of the Parmesan, stirring well to combine. Stir in the pasta, then remove the pan from the heat.
- Serve the chicken pasta with the remaining Parmesan sprinkled over the top and garnished with the chilli flakes, if using, and fresh parsley.

NOTE

If you cannot find the cream I have listed, you can replace it with 60ml single cream and 60ml semi-skimmed milk. Add it over a low heat and gradually increase the heat to stop it curdling. This is meal-prep friendly. It will keep in the fridge for up to four days – loosen the sauce with a tablespoon of water when reheating.

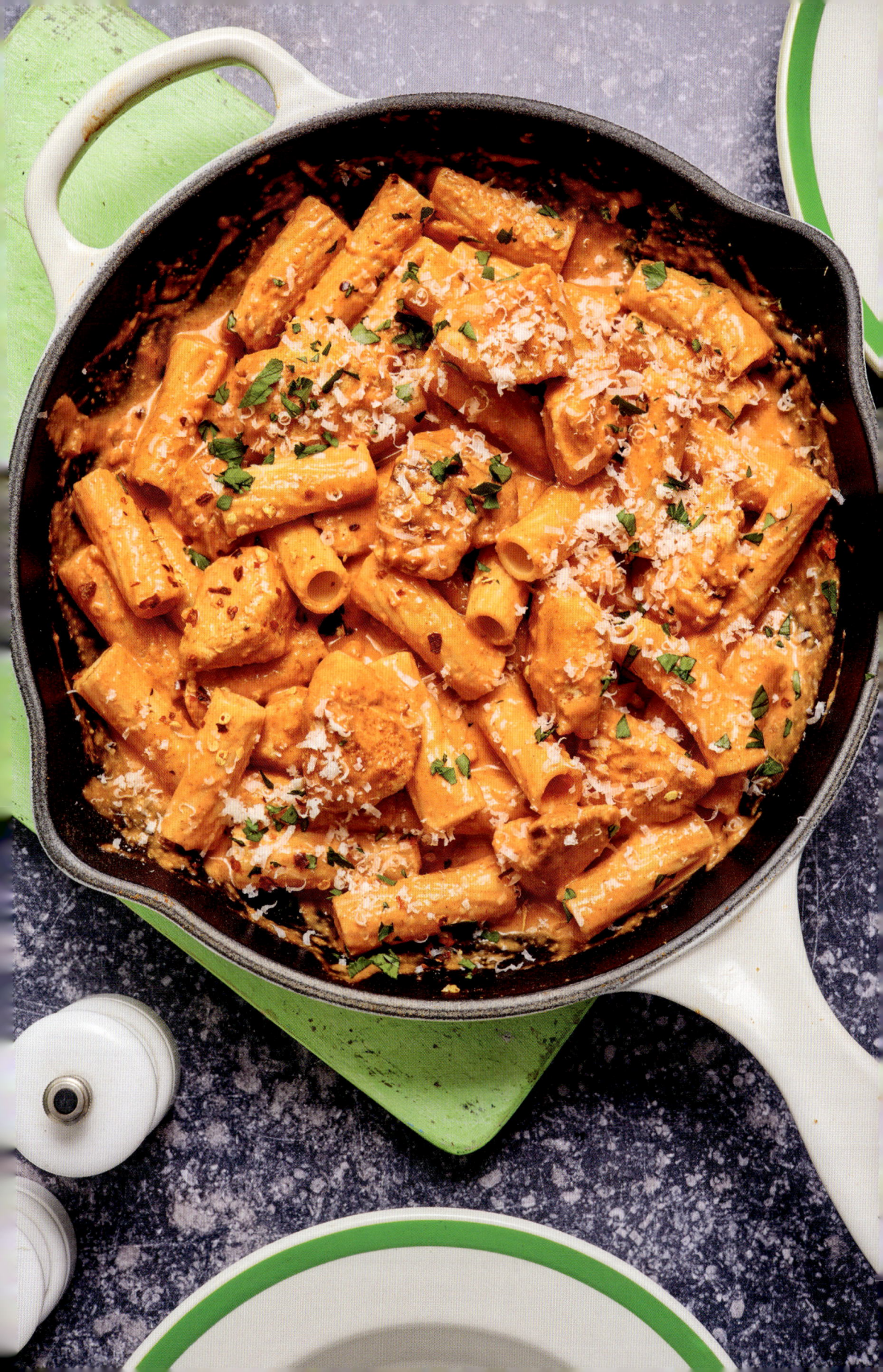

Spanish-Style Chicken with Couscous

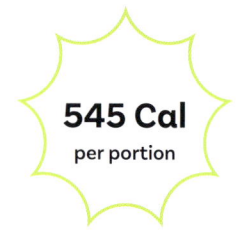

545 Cal per portion

Protein: 46.7g | Fat: 15.4g | Carbs: 44.8g

SERVES 2

This recipe is a nod to my late grandma. When I was younger, she would make this when we went round for tea and it was always one of my favourites. This version uses a homemade Spanish-inspired sauce, along with diced chorizo for added flavour. It also pairs well with golden savoury rice or mashed potato (both ways my gran used to serve it!).

Ingredients

60g chorizo, finely diced
200g skinless chicken breast, cut into 2cm cubes
1 red onion, diced
1 small green pepper, diced
1 small red pepper, diced
1 tsp chopped garlic
½ tsp dried oregano
1½ tsp smoked paprika
1 tsp Italian herb seasoning
1 tbsp tomato purée
1 chicken stock cube
250g tomatoes, finely chopped
100ml boiling water
1 × 110g packet of roasted vegetable couscous
Salt and pepper
A few sprigs of fresh parsley, to garnish

Method

- Start by heating a large frying pan over a medium-high heat. Add the chorizo and cook for 3–4 minutes, until crispy. Remove and set to one side, leaving its oils behind.
- Season the chicken with salt and pepper before adding it to the pan. Cook over a high heat for 6 minutes, then add the onion and peppers.
- Sauté the veggies for 2 minutes, until slightly soft, then add the chopped garlic for 30 seconds. Turn the heat down to medium, then add the dried oregano, smoked paprika and Italian herb seasoning, along with a pinch of salt and pepper.
- Mix the seasonings well to combine, before adding the tomato purée. Crumble over the chicken stock cube before pouring in the chopped tomatoes and water. Leave over a medium heat to simmer for 5 minutes.
- While the chicken simmers, make up the couscous according to the packet instructions.
- Stir half of the chorizo back through the sauce and remove from the heat.
- Serve the couscous along with the chicken and sauce. Top with the remaining chorizo and garnish with fresh parsley.

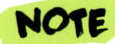

This is meal-prep friendly – it will keep in the fridge for up to four days.

Creamy Tomato Gnocchi

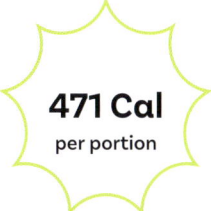

471 Cal per portion

| Protein: 19.7g | Fat: 15.4g | Carbs: 54.9g |

SERVES 2

This is one of those super-easy recipes that never fails to taste banging. Pillowy tender bites of gnocchi are paired with juicy cherry tomatoes in a creamy sauce, topped with mozzarella and basil leaves for a fresh yet comforting dish. Chicken or diced chorizo pair well with this recipe; if you use either you can reduce the gnocchi by 100g.

Ingredients

Olive oil spray
400g fresh gnocchi
1 red onion, diced
150g cherry tomatoes
2 tsp chopped garlic
1½ tbsp tomato purée
1 tsp Italian herb seasoning
200ml hot vegetable stock
50ml semi-skimmed milk
50g light cream cheese
50g mozzarella, grated (or 1 light mozzarella ball, sliced)
Salt and pepper
A few fresh basil leaves, finely sliced, to garnish

Method

- Preheat the grill to high.
- Start by spraying a frying pan with a few pumps of olive oil spray. Add the gnocchi and fry over a high heat for around 5 minutes, until slightly crispy. Remove from the pan and set to one side.
- Add the onion and cherry tomatoes and fry for 4-5 minutes, until the tomatoes start to soften, then add the chopped garlic, stirring for 30 seconds.
- Next, add the tomato purée and herb seasoning along with salt and pepper to taste.
- Turn down the heat, before pouring in the vegetable stock along with the milk and cream cheese. Stir gradually to combine before returning the gnocchi to the pan.
- Turn the heat to medium and leave everything to bubble for a couple of minutes. Remove from the heat before topping with the mozzarella.
- Place the pan under the grill for 4-5 minutes until the cheese is bubbling.
- Remove, and garnish with the fresh basil leaves to serve.

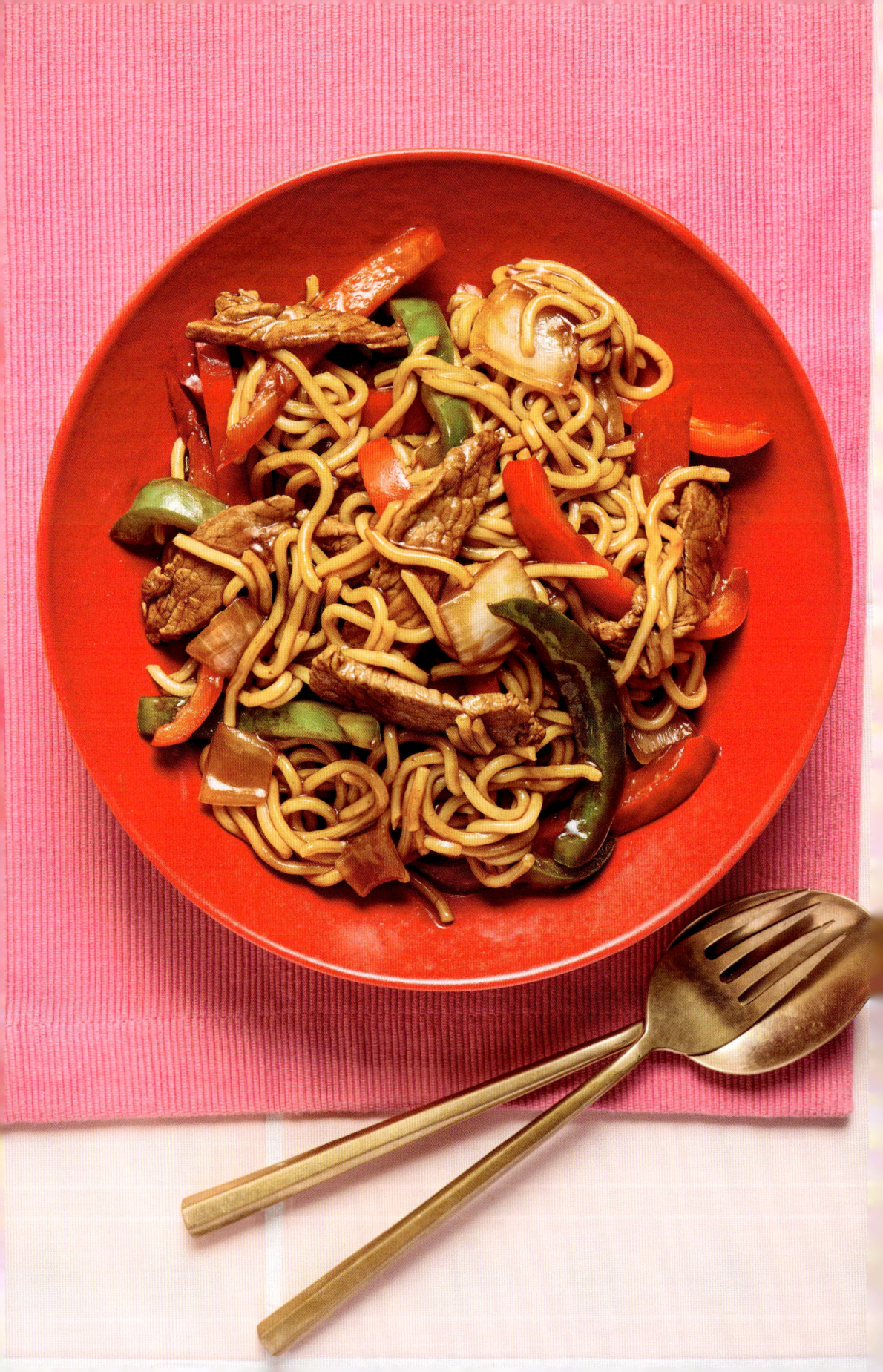

Black Pepper Beef Noodles

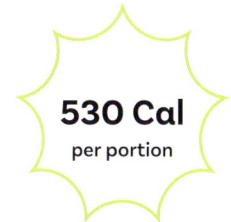

530 Cal per portion

| Protein: 31.1g | Fat: 15.4g | Carbs: 56.4g |

SERVES 2

Once you add these noodles to your weekly rotation there is no going back. For such a fast dinner they really do pack a flavour punch. You can add some extra veggies on the side to bulk it out further, such as pan-fried broccoli or pak choi.

Ingredients

200g steak (either sirloin or other thin variety), cut into thin slices
1½ tsp freshly cracked black pepper
1 tsp sesame oil
1 white onion, cut into chunks
1 red pepper, sliced
1 green pepper, sliced
1 tsp chopped garlic
1 tsp chopped ginger
2 × 150g packets of ready-to-wok medium noodles
Salt

Sauce
200ml hot beef stock
1 tbsp cornflour
2 tbsp dark soy sauce
1 tbsp light soy sauce
2 tbsp oyster sauce
1 tbsp rice wine vinegar

Method

- Start by heating a wok over a high heat.
- While the wok heats, season the steak with 1 teaspoon of the black pepper along with a pinch of salt.
- Add the sesame oil to the wok and, once hot, add the steak. Fry for 3 minutes, then remove from the pan, leaving behind the juices, and set to one side.
- Add the onion, peppers, garlic and ginger and sauté for a few minutes until they are soft.
- While the veggies cook, make the sauce by combining the ingredients in a jug.
- Once the veggies are soft, add the noodles and cook for 2-3 minutes, until soft.
- Pour in the sauce and return the beef to the pan, along with the remaining ½ teaspoon black pepper. Toss to combine and allow the sauce to thicken, which should happen quickly, then remove from the heat.
- Divide equally between two bowls to serve.

Rosemary Garlic Steak with Mash

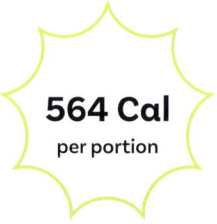
564 Cal per portion

Protein: 35.2g **Fat: 20.6g** **Carbs: 48.3g**

SERVES 2

I think this may be my favourite recipe in the book. It tastes so luxurious yet it's so minimal. I love serving some Chantenay carrots or Tenderstem broccoli with this one, and you can even serve it with crispy potatoes, over rice or with any other carb you prefer.

Ingredients

500g Maris Piper potatoes, cut into 2.5cm cubes

200g rump steak (or any of your choice)

35g light butter

3 sprigs of fresh rosemary

2 tsp chopped garlic

10g plain flour

270ml semi-skimmed milk

15g Parmesan, grated

Salt and pepper

Method

- Start by adding the potatoes to a large pan of salted boiling water. Cook for 14 minutes or until tender when pierced with a fork.
- Meanwhile, season the steak all over with salt and pepper.
- Heat a large pan over a high heat and add 10g of the butter along with the rosemary.
- Add the steak to the pan and cook for 1½ minutes each side, tossing it in the butter, then turn down the heat slightly and add the garlic.
- Flip the steak every 30 seconds for 2 minutes, basting it with the pan juices, for medium-rare. Cook for longer if you prefer your steak well done. Remove from the pan.
- Remove the rosemary sprigs from the pan, turn the heat down to medium and add another 10g of the butter. When it starts to melt, add the flour, stirring continuously with a whisk to form a roux (a thick paste).
- Once a roux has formed, add 200ml of the milk in 50ml increments, whisking continuously.
- Season the roux with salt and pepper, add the grated Parmesan and keep stirring to allow the sauce to thicken while the potatoes finish cooking. If the sauce is bubbling fiercely and thickening quickly, turn the heat down to low.
- Once the potatoes have finished cooking, drain and season with a good pinch of salt and pepper. Add the remaining 15g butter and 70ml milk and mash using a potato masher until smooth.
- Slice the steak into cubes and serve on top of the mashed potatoes. Drizzle over the creamy Parmesan sauce.

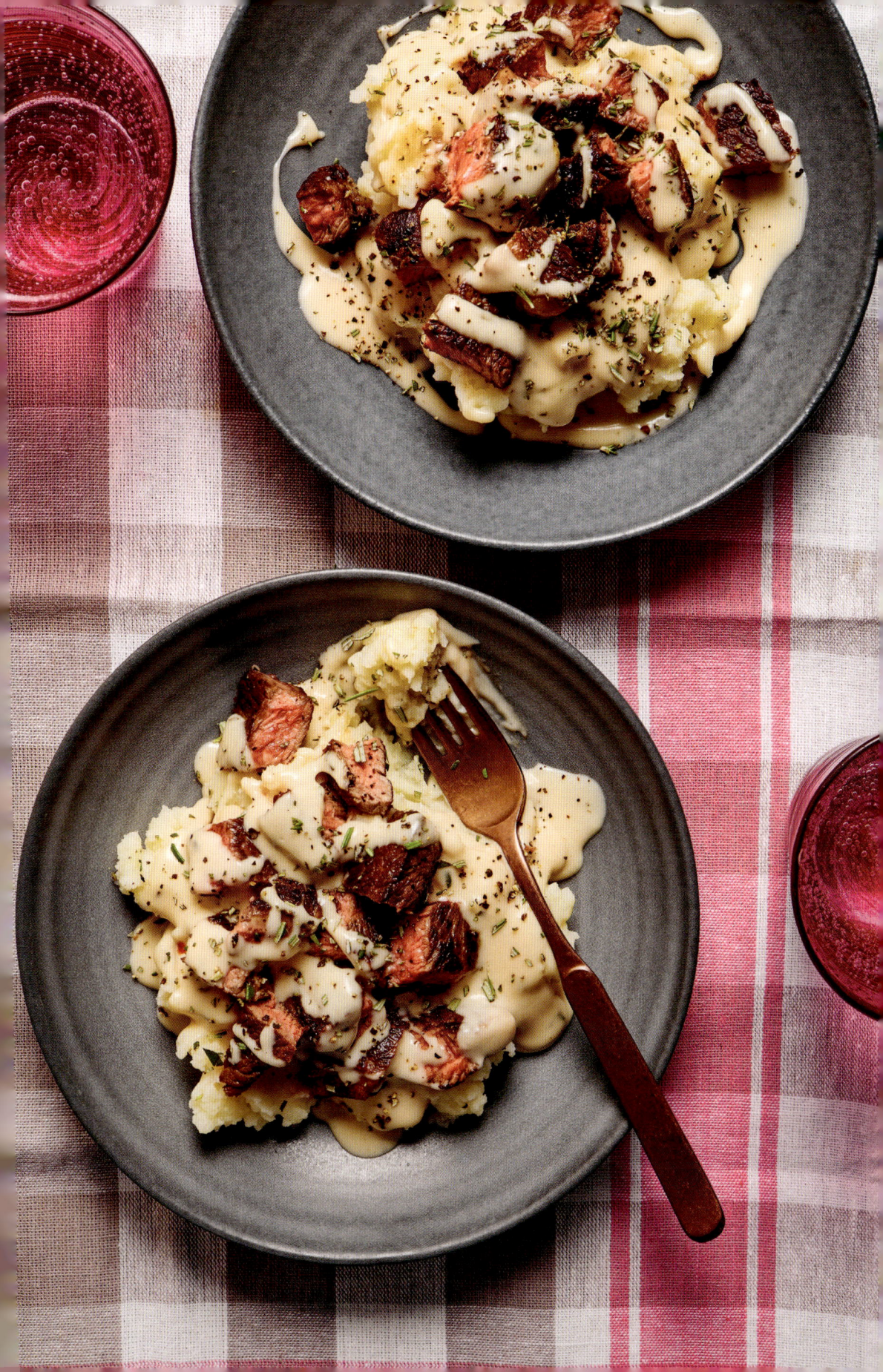

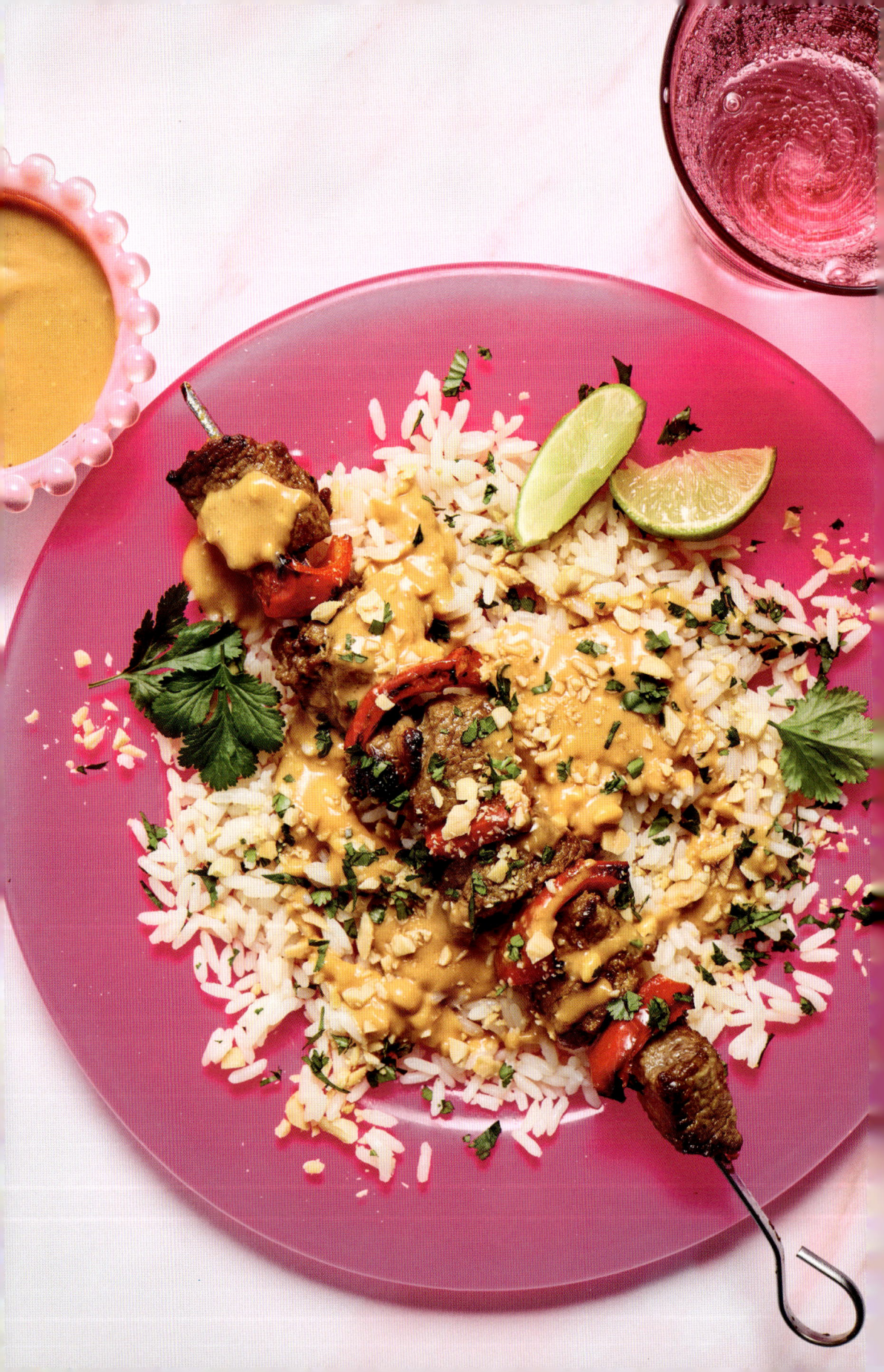

Beef Satay with Peanut Sauce

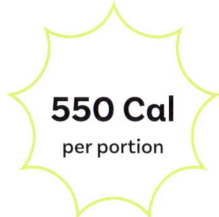

550 Cal per portion

| Protein: 33.6g | Fat: 18.1g | Carbs: 57.3g |

SERVES 2

The beef in this recipe is banging alone, but with the gorgeous peanut sauce drizzled all over it, it's a seriously moreish dish. Make sure that the steak is cooked through, otherwise it will be chewy. Although this recipe can be made in under 20 minutes, I recommend adding marinating time to allow the beef to be the most tender it can be.

Ingredients

1 × 125g packet of boil-in-the-bag rice
200g rump steak, cut into 2.5cm cubes
50ml light coconut milk
1 tsp mild curry powder
1 tsp chopped garlic
½ tbsp red Thai curry paste
1 tsp fish sauce
¼ tsp bicarbonate of soda
¼ tsp salt
1 red pepper, cut into chunks
Neutral cooking spray
5g peanuts, chopped
2 sprigs of fresh coriander, chopped
2 lime wedges (optional)

Peanut sauce
60ml light coconut milk
½ tbsp red Thai curry paste
25g peanut butter
1 tsp brown sugar
1 tsp dark soy sauce
1 tbsp rice wine vinegar
1 tbsp water

Method

- Start by cooking the rice according to the packet instructions.
- Add the cubed steak to a bowl along with the coconut milk, curry powder, garlic, curry paste, fish sauce, bicarbonate of soda and salt. Give it all a good stir and set to one side (see Note).
- In a separate bowl, mix together all of the ingredients for the peanut sauce.
- Thread the steak and red pepper onto small metal skewers. If using wooden skewers, they will need to be cut small to fit in a pan and soaked for 30 minutes prior to use.
- Spray a large frying pan with a few pumps of cooking spray.
- Add each of the skewers to the pan, drizzling over any sauce left from the marinating bowl. Cook for 2½ minutes on each side, for a total of 10 minutes, ensuring the steak is cooked through.
- Meanwhile, pour the peanut sauce into a saucepan and leave over a medium heat to thicken.
- Once the rice is cooked, divide between two bowls. Top with the steak skewers and drizzle over the peanut sauce. Garnish with the chopped peanuts and fresh coriander and serve with the lime wedges, if using.

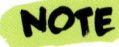

While the bicarbonate of soda helps to tenderise the beef, this recipe works best with marinating time to allow the steak to become really tender – anywhere between 3 and 24 hours is best.

Index

aioli, garlic 143
aubergine 111
   aubergine parmigiana 82
avocado 11, 14, 53
   eggcado breakfast sandwiches 12

bacon 18, 32, 40
   bacon cheeseburger bowls 69
   bacon cheeseburger pasta 124
   baconnaise double cheeseburgers 145
   best ever bacon sandwich 63
   BLT bagels 42
   chicken, bacon and mozzarella pasta 122
bagels, BLT 42
baguettes, chicken gravy stuffing 166
banh mi, bang bang chicken 142
banoffee pie pancake stack 22
béchamel sauce 98
beef
   bacon cheeseburger bowls 69
   bacon cheeseburger pasta 124
   baconnaise double cheeseburgers 145
   beef satay with peanut sauce 189
   black pepper beef noodles 185
   Bolognese potato bake 98
   cheesy chipotle beef pasta 87
   chipotle cheesesteak sub 173
   cottage pie jacket potato 125
   creamy peppercorn steak potatoes 128
   crispy beef quesadillas 50
   crunchwrap supreme 163
   deconstructed enchiladas 170
   feta-stuffed meatballs 73
   garlic aioli steak sandwiches 143
   garlic butter chilli beef tacos 159
   lasagne soup 179
   nacho beef folded wraps 146
   pizza-flavoured stuffed peppers 64
   rosemary garlic steak with mash 186
   Swedish meatballs and mash 78
   taco beef crispy basket bowl 59

Bolognese potato bake 98
bread, cheesy garlic 94
broccoli
   garlic crumb chicken and broccoli bake 101
   pesto chicken and broccoli rice 174
burgers 69, 124, 145
burrito bowls, breakfast 11

'casserole', smoky sausage 94
Cheddar 11, 27, 56, 59–60, 94, 98, 101, 124–5, 143, 146, 159, 169–70, 173
cheese 8, 45, 91, 118, 152
   bacon cheeseburger pasta 124
   baconnaise double cheeseburgers 145
   cheesy chicken and chorizo pasta 91
   cheesy chipotle beef pasta 87
   cheesy garlic bread 94
   cheesy herby salmon and mash 169
   chipotle cheesesteak sub 173
   gochujang garlic bread cheese toastie 70
   ham and cheese puff bakes 60
   see also Cheddar; cream cheese; feta; halloumi; mozzarella; Parmesan; Red Leicester
chicken
   bang bang chicken banh mi 142
   BBQ chicken ranch pasta salad 32
   BBQ shredded chicken Cajun fries 152
   buffalo chicken lettuce wraps 56
   Cajun garlic Parmesan chicken skewers 117
   cheesy chicken and chorizo pasta 91
   chicken, bacon and mozzarella pasta 122
   chicken Caesar salad pitta breads 40
   chicken gravy stuffing baguettes 166
   chicken mushroom 'pot noodle' 46
   chicken Parm pasta 175

chicken shawarma flatbreads 153
chicken tikka buns 139
chipotle chicken fajitas 118
creamy Parmesan Cajun chicken and rice 92
crispy chicken snack wraps 45
crispy orange chicken 160
garlic crumb chicken and broccoli bake 101
gochujang chicken pasta 180
Greek-style chicken orzo 99
lemon pepper chicken 110
naked chicken kebab 41
pad Thai-style noodles 131
peri chicken pasta salad jars 39
pesto chicken and broccoli rice 174
saucy Korean-style chicken with brown rice 176
Singapore-style noodles 93
Spanish-style chicken with couscous 182
spicy chicken pizza wrap 55
spicy chicken sliders 115
sticky chorizo stuffed chicken 121
sticky gochujang chicken flatbreads 155
sticky sesame chicken on noodles 88
sweet chilli glazed chicken bites 85
Tandoori chicken rice bowls 86
Thai sweet chilli chicken tenders 116
chickpea spicy pitta breads 35
chocolate chip brioche French toast bites 28
chorizo 112, 182
   cheesy chicken and chorizo pasta 91
   egg and chorizo hash browns 25
   sticky chorizo stuffed chicken 121
cottage pie jacket potato 125
couscous 106, 182
cream cheese 15, 70, 78, 91, 101, 121, 169, 174, 183
curry, halloumi 76

egg 18, 93
- egg and chorizo hash browns 25
- eggcado breakfast sandwiches 12
- Hollandaise over eggs 20
- omelette 27
- sausage and egg muffins 8
- scrambled oat bowl 26
- spinach, egg and feta wrap 15

enchiladas, deconstructed 170

fajitas, chipotle chicken 118
feta 99
- feta-stuffed meatballs 73
- spinach, egg and feta wrap 15

fish
- Baja-style fish tacos 109
- lemon pepper mayo fish finger butty 66
- lemon pepper Parmesan fish and chips 149
- tuna sushi bowls 53
- *see also* salmon

flatbreads
- chicken shawarma 153
- gochujang chicken 155
- halloumi souvlaki 111
- margherita pesto 65

French toast bites 28
full English shakshuka 18
gnocchi, creamy tomato 183
gravy, onion 127
gyoza noodle bowls 140

halloumi 39
- halloumi curry 76
- halloumi souvlaki flatbreads 111
- hot honey halloumi tacos 156
- sweet chilli halloumi salad 36, 37

ham 27
- ham and cheese puff bakes 60

hash browns, egg and chorizo 25
Hollandaise over eggs 20

kebabs
- lamb shish 150
- naked chicken 41

lamb shish kebabs 150
lasagne soup 179
lettuce 32, 39, 40, 45, 59, 66, 69, 86, 145, 146, 153, 155, 163
- BLT bagels 42
- buffalo chicken lettuce wraps 56

margherita pesto flatbread 65
mash 78, 127, 169, 186
mayo
- garlic 139
- gochujang mayo sauce 155

meatballs 73, 78
mozzarella 50, 54, 55, 65, 70, 82, 87, 115, 121, 139, 179, 183
- chicken, bacon and mozzarella pasta 122

muffins 20
- sausage and egg 8

mushroom 18
- chicken mushroom 'pot noodle' 46

nacho beef folded wraps 146
noodles
- black pepper beef noodles 185
- chicken mushroom 'pot noodle' 46
- pad Thai-style noodles 131
- Singapore-style noodles 93
- sticky sesame chicken on noodles 88
- vegetable gyoza noodle bowls 140

oat(s) 17
- scrambled oat bowl 26

omelette, 'on the go' 27
onion
- onion gravy 127
- sumac onions 153

pad Thai-style noodles 131
pancakes, banoffee pie 22
panko breadcrumbs 66, 73, 78, 82, 101, 106, 149, 175
Parmesan 40, 42, 70, 101, 106, 128, 149, 169, 174, 175, 179, 180, 186
- Cajun garlic Parmesan chicken skewers 117
- chicken Parm pasta 175
- creamy Parmesan Cajun chicken and rice 92

passata 64, 82, 175, 179
pasta
- bacon cheeseburger pasta 124
- BBQ chicken ranch pasta salad 32
- cheesy chicken and chorizo pasta 91
- cheesy chipotle beef pasta 87
- chicken, bacon and mozzarella pasta 122
- chicken Parm pasta 175

chilli garlic prawn linguine 112
gochujang chicken pasta 180
Greek-style chicken orzo 99
lasagne soup 179
peri chicken pasta salad jars 39

peanut sauce 189
pepper 11, 39, 87, 93, 94, 99, 102, 118, 150, 170, 173, 182, 185
- lemon pepper mayo fish finger butty 66
- pizza-flavoured stuffed peppers 64

pesto 82
- margherita pesto flatbread 65
- pesto chicken and broccoli rice 174

pickled vegetables 142
pitta breads
- chicken Caesar salad 40
- spicy chickpea 35

pizza
- pizza-flavoured stuffed peppers 64
- spicy chicken pizza wrap 55

pork
- gochujang BBQ pork bowls 81
- sweet and sticky pork fried rice 96

potato 11, 69
- Bolognese potato bake 98
- creamy peppercorn steak potatoes 128
- honey BBQ sausage and potatoes 102
- mash 78, 127, 169, 186
- speedy cottage pie jacket potato 125

prawn linguine, chilli garlic 112
puff bakes, ham and cheese 60

quesadillas, crispy beef 50

raspberry 28
- white chocolate raspberry breakfast crumbles 17

Red Leicester 32, 56, 69, 87, 91, 170
rice
- beef satay with peanut sauce 189
- creamy Parmesan Cajun chicken and rice 92
- crispy orange chicken 160
- firecracker salmon 132
- gochujang BBQ pork bowls 81
- halloumi curry 76
- pesto chicken and broccoli rice 174

rice (cont.)
  pizza-flavoured stuffed peppers 64
  salmon yakitori 136
  saucy Korean-style chicken with brown rice 176
  spicy tuna sushi bowls 53
  sweet chilli glazed chicken bites 85
  sweet and sticky pork 96
  Tandoori chicken rice bowls 86

salads 41, 60, 156
  BBQ chicken ranch pasta salad 32
  chicken Caesar salad pitta breads 40
  peri chicken pasta salad jars 39
  sweet chilli halloumi salad 36, 37
salmon
  cheesy herby salmon and mash 169
  crunchy garlic butter salmon bites with couscous 106
  firecracker salmon 132
  salmon yakitori 136
sandwiches
  best ever bacon 63
  eggcado breakfast 12
  garlic aioli steak 143
  lemon pepper mayo fish finger butty 66
satay beef with peanut sauce 189

sauces 11, 45, 66, 78, 85, 88, 93, 106, 110, 132, 160, 176, 185
  béchamel 98
  burger 69, 124
  Caesar 40
  chipotle 63, 109
  chive 25
  garlic 153, 156
  garlic aioli 143
  garlic and coriander 86
  garlic herb 73
  garlic herb yoghurt 36
  garlic yoghurt 41
  gochujang mayo 155
  Hollandaise 20
  pad Thai-style 131
  peanut 189
  peri 39
sausage 11, 18
  bangers and mash with onion gravy 127
  honey BBQ sausage and potatoes 102
  sausage and egg muffins 8
  smashed sausage tacos 14
  smoky sausage 'casserole' with cheesy garlic bread 94
shakshuka, full English 18
soup lasagne 54, 179
spinach 12, 76, 179
  spinach, egg and feta wrap 15
sushi bowls, spicy tuna 53
sweetcorn 32, 46, 59

tacos
  Baja-style fish 109
  garlic butter chilli beef 159
  hot honey halloumi 156
  smashed sausage 14
  taco beef crispy basket bowl 59
toastie, gochujang garlic bread cheese 70
tomato 11, 12, 15, 18, 25, 27, 32, 36, 41, 60, 63, 65, 69, 76, 94, 98, 99, 109, 111, 112, 153, 159, 163, 174, 182
  BLT bagels 42
  creamy tomato gnocchi 183
  speedy tomato soup 54
tortilla chips 45, 146, 163
  tortilla wraps 14–15, 45, 50, 55, 59, 109, 118, 146, 156, 159, 163, 170
tuna sushi bowls 53

vegetable gyoza noodle bowls 140
vegetables, quick pickled 142

white chocolate raspberry breakfast crumbles 17
wraps
  buffalo chicken lettuce 56
  crispy chicken 45
  crunchwrap supreme 163
  nacho beef 146
  spicy chicken pizza 55
  spinach, egg and feta 15

Acknowledgements

To start, I owe a huge thank you to Ru Merritt for believing in me and for giving me another opportunity. To Liv Nightingall, my editor, for your patience and support in this book coming together, and to Francesca Thomson, who has been my uplifter and motivator whenever I've needed it. For all those involved in the visuals; Ellis Parrinder, Troy Willis, Rosie Reynolds and Daisy Shayler-Webb, just when I thought the photos couldn't get any better, you outdo yourselves and breathe such life into the recipes. To Michelle and Rosie at Studio Noel for designing yet another remarkable cover and to Nicky Barneby for the stunning internals. To my family, thank you for your love, patience and continued support.

Finally, thank you for grabbing a copy of my book and allowing me to fulfil my passion. Words cannot express my gratitude to each and every one of you who supports me. I hope this book shows you just how much you can enjoy the food that you love (even on a time limit) and still reach where you want to be.